COMMUNICATION STRATEGIES FOR PEOPLE WITH DEVELOPMENTAL DISABILITIES

COMMUNICATION STRATEGIES FOR PEOPLE WITH DEVELOPMENTAL DISABILITIES

Issues from Theory and Practice

General Editor:

Ken Linfoot PhD

Charles Sturt University-Mitchell
Bathurst, NSW, Australia

·P A U L·H·
BROOKES
PUBLISHING Co

Baltimore . London . Toronto . Sydney

Paul H. Brookes Publishing Co.
PO Box 10624
Baltimore, Maryland 21285-0624

Printed and bound in Australia

Library of Congress Cataloging-in-Publication Data

Communication strategies for people with developmental disabilities:
issues from theory and practice/general editor, Ken Linfoot.
p. cm.
Includes bibliographical references and index.

ISBN 1-55766-170-7: $33.00

1. Developmentally disabled children—Education—Research.
2. Developmentally disabled—Education—Research. 3. Communicative disorders—Patients—Education—Research. I. Linfoot, Ken.
LC4601.C63 1994
371.91′4—dc20 93-50222
CIP

Contents

Notes on the Contributors

Michael Arthur trained as a primary (or elementary) school teacher at Macquarie University in Sydney, New South Wales, before working in both special and regular schools as a teacher of students who experience mild, moderate or severe intellectual disability. Following completion of an MA (Special Education) at Macquarie University, he taught for a number of years before taking up a lectureship in special education at Charles Sturt University-Mitchell in Bathurst, New South Wales. During this time Michael directed his research to the needs of personnel working with students and others who have a severe disability, especially in the area of communication interventions.

Michael is currently lecturing in special education at the University of Newcastle and completing a PhD in the area of behaviour state in people who experience the most severe disabilities. Other research interests include educational change processes, especially in relation to integration, behaviour management and the role of support services such as respite care.

Nancy Butterfield completed initial teacher training at Armidale Teachers College in New South Wales and received the Diploma in Teaching and Graduate Diploma in Educational Studies (Special Education) from Charles Sturt University-Mitchell, where she is currently completing the MEd by research on communication abilities of students with severe intellectual disability.

Her professional experience has included teaching students with moderate and severe intellectual disability, serving as Director of an Early Intervention Program, lecturing in special education to trainee teachers, serving as a Research Associate to a project on communication skills development, as Regional Adviser on the integration of students with disabilities and as Senior Educational Officer for the Early Learning Program with the New South Wales Department of School Education.

Nancy's research and professional interests include language development, non-verbal communication and early intervention issues for students with disabilities, within the context of integrated educational placement alternatives.

Kathleen Dice received BA and BEd degrees from the University of Saskatchewan at Saskatoon, Canada. She subsequently completed a Graduate Diploma in Educational Studies (Special Education) at Charles Sturt University-Mitchell.

Kathleen's background is that of a classroom and remedial teacher. She has worked in primary (or elementary) schools in both Canada and Australia. Within the field of special education, Kathleen's particular interests are remedial teaching, learning disabilities and non-speech communication.

Presently, she is employed as a teacher of children with severe and moderate intellectual disability at Kempsey West Public School Support Unit in New South Wales.

Sue Healy has had extensive experience as a special educator in settings ranging from early childhood to high schools. Her training included a Diploma in Teaching (Early Childhood) from the Institute of Early Childhood in Melbourne, Victoria, a BEd from the University of Canberra in the Australian Capital Territory and a Graduate Diploma in Educational Studies (Special Education) from Charles Sturt University-Mitchell.

As Executive Teacher and Deputy Principal at Koomarri Special School in Canberra for over ten years, Sue was particularly interested in assisting the development of communication in students with disabilities. She is now Principal of Cranleigh Special School in the Australian Capital Territory.

Ken Linfoot holds BA, MLitt and MEd degrees from the University of New England in New South Wales and received a PhD in special education from Macquarie University. His initial teacher training was at Bathurst Teachers College. He has worked as a teacher in regular and special education and as a school counsellor and district guidance officer with the New South Wales Department of Education.

Ken is currently Senior Lecturer in Special Education at Charles Sturt University-Mitchell and Director of the Special Education Centre. He is responsible for special education and school counselling courses at undergraduate and post-graduate levels as well as the operation of an Early Intervention Project located on the university campus; he has also directed a number of research and development projects involving services for children with intellectual disabilities. His research interests involve communication disorders, issues in early intervention services and access to special education for students in rural and isolated areas. He is currently Editor of *The Australasian Journal of Special Education*.

Diana Messervy obtained her initial Diploma in Teaching (Early Childhood) from Brisbane Kindergarten Teachers College in Queensland. Since then she has worked in a variety of early childhood and primary (or elementary) school settings in Australia and the United States. These have included community kindergartens, a preschool distance education program, a resource program for students with learning disabilities and a community-based preschool early intervention program. Diana has taught at the College of Technical and Further Education in Cairns, Queensland, where she was involved in personnel preparation for work in day care and early childhood settings. In 1990 she completed a Graduate Diploma in Educational Studies (Special Education) at Charles Sturt University-Mitchell.

She has particular interest in the language and social skill development of young children with intellectual disability. This resulted in part from her work with a multidisciplinary team involved in integrating children with special needs into early childhood centres.

She is currently Teaching Director at Bayview Heights Community Kindergarten in Cairns, Queensland.

Foreword

James Ward

Formerly Professor of Special Education and Director,
Centre for Research into Special Education and Rehabilitation
Macquarie University, Sydney, NSW

Recently I had the privilege of watching a well-trained teacher of young children at work: she was engaged in teaching language and communication skills to John, a five year old with Down syndrome. By any standards her performance was exemplary. Training proceeded in a relaxed and natural way, with frequent contingent praise: the content of the lesson, the use of communicative forms related entirely to what the child was doing in a play situation. He was attentive and motivated throughout. An outstanding feature of the teacher's technique was her attempt to obtain generalisation. Thus the same forms were practised with a variety of materials, in different parts of the room and with children and other adults present, including the child's mother and an aide. In the course of an hour the teacher modelled a variety of communicative behaviours, for different children, using greater complexity of language and a longer mean length of utterance when appropriate. Afterwards the reasons for all this were explained to the adults who observed the session and who, like me I must say, were very impressed. However, John used very few examples of spontaneous or elaborate language. His best effort appeared to be a three-word utterance "Me want gun."

It was now time for gross motor activities in a somewhat restricted play area. John was driving a pedal car which brought him into violent contact with a tricycle ridden by Paul. John was very cross "Po get out way — me drive". Paul declined to move. Once again "Po get out way", this time in a scream. The aide decided that it was time to avoid the impending conflict and removed John for toileting. But when they returned a fresh conflict arose, as Paul had abandoned his tricycle and had taken over John's pedal car. "Po — me want red car" etc. At this point John's mother intervened and prevented another fracas. She told me that John talked a great deal at home but that the family could not understand much of what he tried to say. However, at all times they acted as if they did.

I tell this story to illustrate two points: the relative normality of John's behaviour and the improvement in his pragmatic use of language in the natural setting of a playground and his peer group. Undoubtedly some articulation training would help but, provided that the present favourable circumstances continue, the prognosis for John to develop adequate linguistic skills, even without further interventions, is probably very good.

However, for many persons of comparable ability the situation has always been vastly different. I think now of Bill, a man with intellectual disability, who has been institutionalised since the age of five. The hospital has for many years provided fairly sophisticated programs for language and communication, mainly for educational reasons but also to contribute to a well organised process of de-institutionalisation. In the course of these programs Bill has developed a limited spoken vocabulary and receptive language skills. Ostensibly he is a prime candidate for living in the open community.

The problem is, however, that the skills Bill has painfully acquired in the course of the education program transfer only minimally to situations like recreation and the cafeteria, and are hardly relevant in the place in which I would think that they were most useful, the residential accommodation. Clearly he has learned some sort of discrimination between various settings from which he does not appear to be able to escape. In addition the problem is compounded by social interactions of the most basic kind, e.g. Bill's arm waving or "hi" being intermittently reinforced by other patients and the staff. Here we have a sort of behavioural trap: if the basic attempts at communication are ignored, they will certainly be reinforced by others. Thus the social use of language is being maintained at a low level. A way out of this situation might be for those with whom Bill interacts to insist upon more normal pragmatic exchanges, standing reasonably close, maintaining eye contact, etc. Although time-consuming, such obvious cueing could provide better transfer of linguistic skills from one context to another. But much of the time Bill would find such exchanges aversive.

Even so, and despite the presence of severe disability, both Bill and John have functional communication systems, which includes spoken language. However, there are many disabled persons for whom the development of a communication system of any sort must take precedence over training in language. I think now of Jill, a twelve-year-old girl showing not only severe retardation but serious auditory and visual impairments. Jill was institutionalised at the age of two on the advice of a pediatrician who considered that the family would no longer be able to cope with her now that there was a new baby, adding to the three other siblings. Once Jill entered a special school a great deal of time was devoted to attempts to teach her a simple spoken vocabulary and, when those failed, a repertoire of manual signs. There was some success in the latter area but this was eventually dissipated by the tendency of some teachers and caregivers to accept any vague approximation to a sign rather than insisting upon precision. The parents, who visited regularly and had gone to the trouble of learning signs so that Jill could return home at weekends, were understandably frustrated. However, a remarkable breakthrough occurred when the staff decided to restrict their efforts to teaching Jill to use a simple 25-item picture communication board which allowed her to communicate her basic needs within the school. This was immediately successful, with the result that a second board for use in a nearby shopping centre was devised. This worked equally well. The fact that Jill now had a basic form of communication had a marked effect upon her parents, who were now happy for her to stay with them over weekends and holidays. What was even less predictable was that Jill began to replace the first communication board with signs and, in one or two cases, spoken words. She now presents a totally different picture, is more sociable and is making what, for her, is rapid progress in schoolwork.

Jill's case has unusual features but in general it illustrates the fact that, provided teachers and caregivers have patience and willingness to experiment, even multiply-handicapped children can acquire a functional system of augmented communication. There are others, however, for whom the eventual acquisition of communicative skills is highly idiosyncratic. A particular example was Don, a ten-year-old boy attending a school for multiply-handicapped students.

Don was profoundly hearing-impaired with considerable visual impairment except in the immediate visual field. He also had moderate mobility problems. Because of these disabilities it was possible to make only a speculative assessment of his potential, but he was considered to have severe intellectual disability. Since Don had some degree of usable vision it was natural that attempts were made to teach him conventional signing and initially he acquired about thirty signs. Unfortunately, however, by the time he was eight there was no further progress: he had reached a plateau in his development of communication skills although in other areas, like self-help and fine motor skills, he had made steady progress.

Attempts were made to solve the problem with a program of intensive signing, combined as necessary with use of a communication board, but major progress only occurred when, by chance, it was discovered that Don was happiest with the print medium for communication. Through discrimination training he rapidly acquired a functional vocabulary of printed words and was able to communicate his wants by printing out words and, later, phrases. All this had a remarkably positive effect upon Don's behaviour and the ways in which he was perceived by parents, caregivers and teachers.

I cite these cases to illustrate the extreme difficulties and complexities involved in teaching language and communication skills to persons with developmental disabilities, particularly if they have additional disabilities or have been deprived of experience as a consequence of family rejection or institutionalisation. John and Bill represent the powerful effects of context upon communicative behaviour: in Bill's case, its influence upon generalisation or transfer. It is a perennial source of wonder to me that language, which has such obvious survival importance for vulnerable persons, may not be maintained without continual reinforcement or may not transfer across situations. In different ways Jill and Don are examples of the importance of long term and creative teaching, without which neither would have acquired a functional communication system with its power to influence environment. (Incidentally, I have strong doubts as to whether this would have happened in a mainstream classroom). These children also epitomise the idiosyncratic nature of the development of a communication mode in persons with multiple sensory and physical disabilities.

A contemplation of these various problems brings me to the book edited by Dr Linfoot. Here I must confess to a longstanding personal interest both in its subject matter and, at a somewhat more trivial level, in the use of the term "developmental disability" in the title. Public Law 94-142 is internationally well known as a piece of pioneering legislation, but it could be argued that Public Law 94-103, which introduced the concept of developmental disability, was at least as significant for its commitment to lifelong service delivery and for its functional definitions of the main problems faced by the target populations.

A lack of adequate communication strategies is one of the most important problems. Inadequacies in this area are a prime cause of social and educational marginality, failure to achieve independent living and what, for most of us, would be a lifestyle of poor quality: such problems have, of course, been brought into sharp focus by the current movements towards normalisation and mainstreaming. Thus it is now necessary for caregivers, teachers and other professionals to be much better informed than would have been the case twenty years ago. However, this is a complex and ever-changing area of practice, deriving concepts and strategies from many sources: developmental psycholinguistics, abnormal child psychology, instructional theories, experience of using augmented communication, developments in advanced forms of prosthesis, particularly electronic, etc. Unfortunately the implications of this diverse information for actual practice are not always clear.

In these circumstances it is timely that Ken Linfoot and his colleagues have produced a book which examines a range of the strategies involved in developing communication skills in people with developmental disabilities, and have reviewed some of the theoretical and practical issues to which they give rise. Having lived through (or perhaps endured) some of the changes in psycholinguistics which have occurred over the last thirty years, I was particularly interested in some of the remarks in Ken Linfoot's introductory chapter. He points out the importance of the work of Bloom, McLean and Snyder-McLean and others who, in my view, were largely responsible for freeing the field from the somewhat arid and doctrinaire use of operant models which had been central in the 1960s and the early 1970s. They set the scene for the heavy emphasis on pragmatics which is now dominant. However, linguists such as Michael Halliday were also to have a major impact upon the vast expansion of research and publication which occurred in the 1980s, and which was probably best exemplified by the prolific output of Schiefelbusch and his colleagues at the University of Kansas.

An important component of research into developmental disability has been the inclusion of concepts from developmental psychology. These have been especially useful in the area of early intervention, which has had a major impact not only upon behaviour but on community attitudes. Thus in Chapter 2 Nancy Butterfield discusses the use of play as a strategy for both assessment and intervention, referring to a small scale research which explored issues surrounding parallel developments in play and language in six severely intellectually disabled children. If we accept Piaget's theory, play and language both relate to the semiotic function which develops in infancy, partially as a means of coping with the imbalance of assimilation over accommodation during this period. For children with deviant or delayed language the observation of play behaviour can, therefore, be highly instructive. Butterfield's six cases illustrate some of the individual discrepancies between play and language competencies which can occur in young children at comparable developmental levels. The "play" data were obtained through the use of a scale devised by Westby. Among some of the strategies to which reference is made is the "incidental teaching" method of Hart and Risley, which sits well with modern naturalistic and pragmatic approaches to language and communication.

My experience has been that persons with mild intellectual disabilities often possess a diffidence or lack of assertiveness which can handicap them at work and in social situations with peers. Training to overcome this does not always have the desired effect, since a decision to be assertive usually requires a subtle social judgement. Early evidence of this problem is present in the account of a very detailed study presented by Messervy in Chapter 3. Messervy looked at one aspect of pragmatics: requesting behaviour in groups with mild developmental disability, and normal peers. The task was to request a toy from peers in dyadic and group situations. The data showed some interesting, though perhaps predictable, trends in that there was evidence of a general lack of assertiveness in the group with developmental disabilities, and an effect of group size. Messervy canvasses a number of explanations for these and examines ways in which the situation might be improved; modelling appropriate body language, puppetry, etc. For me what most emerged, however, was a very powerful indirect argument in favour of integrated preschools — I would also apply this to the study in Chapter 2.

A problem frequently encountered in teaching severely disabled persons is the choice of an appropriate vocabulary for use in manual signing programs. This is the topic of Chapter 4, a very informative and comprehensive account by Kathleen Dice. The author looks at the main kinds of knowledge which should be applied: developmental, functional and motoric. Dice discusses a wide range of interesting points and criteria, including the issues of translucency and transparency in iconic signs, motoric problems in sign production and ecological considerations. Among the many issues which took my eye was that of obtaining combinations of signs as more complex syntactic forms. Presumably the achievement of two sign combinations can herald a more generative stage in the subject's communications, but in the past I have never found it to be easy. The best tribute I can pay this chapter is to say that I wish that I had been able to refer to it ten years ago!

The issue of context is also dealt with in Ken Linfoot's contribution in Chapter 5. As in the cases of Chapters 2 and 3, the topic is illustrated by reference to a research study. Linfoot reviews a number of studies which have addressed the development of pragmatic forms in both normal and disabled children. In different ways these attempt to identify and categorise the pragmatic features of communication. The review also indicates the importance of context upon these aspects of language use. The actual study was undertaken with sixteen children with severe intellectual disability, most of whom had been institutionalised for long periods. The data for eight of these were subjected to detailed analyses of verbal and non-verbal behaviour recorded from videotaped observations. There were indications of differences between the use of pragmatic forms between children at various developmental levels and also differences between three levels of structure in classroom activities. Referring to the latter point, Linfoot points out the need for environments which minimise adult social control and provide socially interactive settings; inevitably I thought of my first case, Bill. This is an important study which contains a wealth of thought-provoking findings.

High level technology is now having an increasingly powerful impact upon the field of developmental disability, particularly with those with cerebral palsy and physical impairments. For example, a recent search for references to the use of simulation as a training device revealed a host of complex multimedia applications and some more esoteric examples featuring the technology of virtual reality. Referring to rather less ambitious approaches, in Chapter 6 Sue Healy describes the use of a synthetic speech output communication aid (ScanWolf VOCA) with Stephen, a boy with the multiple disabilities of quadriplegia, cerebral palsy and intellectual disability. Considerable observational data indicated improvements in both inititiations of communication and responses to those of others. However, despite rapid improvements in the technology, the use of such an approach clearly demands a great deal of training, both of the target person and those with whom he or she is expected to interact. This is a very useful chapter with a good review of the field of augmented communication. Problems with speech are, of course, common among those with developmental disability, but on reading this chapter I found my thoughts turning to an equally vulnerable group — stroke victims.

In Chapter 7 Arthur provides a thoughtful review of a wide range of contemporary researchers and relates their findings to a three-part cyclical model: individual functioning, immediate social contexts and wider social contexts. Having spent over thirty years in various attempts at change agentry I can empathise with one of his early points: "It cannot be assumed that a knowledge of best practices will automatically result in their implementation". However, it is clear from his discussion that the field of communication is now comfortably eclectic and sensible, without the domination of operant models that occurred in the 1960s and 1970s. To some extent this change has been the result of input from more sophisticated psycholinguistic theories, but in my view the main stimulus has been the failure to produce generalisation effects noted earlier. Arthur raises many issues, one of which might be termed the definition and creation of facilitative communication environments. This is the theme of the final chapter by three of the contributors, Butterfield, Linfoot and Arthur.

Chapter 8 is devoted to practical guidelines for developing communication skills in naturally occurring settings, using strategies to be applied by significant communication partners such as parents, relatives and teachers. The excellent point is made that much of the aberrant and idiosyncratic behaviour of persons with developmental disability represents their attempts to communicate. In describing the development of functional communication, the writers refer to the three stages of pre-intentional, intentional and symbolic forms, which are summarised in a useful table. The production of goals and objectives for intervention results from a process of assessment that uses a wide variety of information sources, including a form of applied behaviour analysis. A conventional sequence of programming steps is described, along with strategies for moving clients up to the next communicative level, e.g. pre-intentional to intentional. The need to perceive communication as a transactional process is reiterated, as is the importance of teaching communication in a coordinated and systematic way.

The foregoing has skipped lightly over some of the content of what is undoubtedly a well written and informative book. Its subject is enormously important, especially in an era of de-institutionalisation and mainstreaming: at the present time we may not be able to maximise cognitive and educational growth for all persons with disabilities but we can, to a much greater extent, develop in many the skills needed for communication and social integration. Dr Linfoot and his colleagues have offered this challenge, together with some up-to-date concepts and strategies by which it can be met by practitioners. I commend them for their efforts and trust that the book will find a ready readership among students, teachers and other professionals with interests in this field.

Chapter 1

Communicative Behaviour in the Least Restrictive Environment

Ken Linfoot

Charles Sturt University-Mitchell
Bathurst, NSW

At a recent meeting of special education teachers, one of the senior participants commented on the newly introduced policy of promoting the integration of children with moderate and severe intellectual disabilities. For some years a regular school had included a special education unit where children with intellectual disabilities could be enrolled, thus allowing the closure of the special school that had catered for those children up to that time. But now it was time to go further. Enrolling children with severe disabilities in the regular school had been a significant step at the time, but it was beginning to be realised that many of the features of education in a special school were still practised in the special education unit in this regular school. After all, if the advantages of normalisation (Wolfensberger, 1972) were to have a chance to benefit these school students, then further opportunities for interaction and learning with normally developing children would have to be found. The teachers and parents at this particular primary (or elementary) school decided to disband the special education class that had been formed for the youngest children (four- to six-year-olds) and to place those children in a number of age-appropriate regular classes within the school. Importantly, the teacher and teacher's aide who were released from the special class by this arrangement were then used to provide in-class support to their former students in their new locations and, of course, to the teachers who had now accepted those children into their regular classes.

The significance of that experience to the subject of this book was demonstrated by the excitement and enthusiasm of the teachers at the school as they spoke of the rapid changes they were noticing in the language and communication abilities of those children. Those who had shown limited ranges of social and communicative behaviour became interested in interacting with other children in their new classes. Moreover, improvements were noticed in the linguistic forms being used by the children. Teachers reported that limited increases in vocabulary usage were becoming apparent and that the children's articulation seemed to be easier to understand.

Clearly, this anecdote is open to many sources of unreliability as evidence of growth in language skills following educational integration or mainstreaming. A complex research design would need to be developed to collect reliable and valid evidence on the association between school placement and educational outcome. However, what is of interest here is that a number of teachers at that school were so impressed with the way in which their new educational strategies were working for students with severe intellectual disabilities that there was at least the perception that student outcomes were improving. Importantly, the improvement for these children was perceived to be in the critical domain of *communication*.

An Inclusionary View of Service Delivery

Services for individuals with developmental disability have altered dramatically in recent years in most Western countries. The writings of Nirje (1970) and Wolfensberger (1972) have resulted in many changes in the ways in which health, education and welfare services have been delivered to this population. These changes are reflected in the commonly accepted view, drawn from a report to the United States Congress (quoted in McDonnell, Wilcox & Hardman, 1991, p 2), which defines developmental disability as:

> a severe, chronic disability of a person which:
>
> (a) is attributable to a mental or physical impairment or combination of mental and physical impairments;
> (b) is manifested before the person attains age twenty-two;
> (c) is likely to continue indefinitely;
> (d) results in substantial functional limitation in three or more of the following areas of major life activity: (i) self-care, (ii) receptive and expressive language, (iii) learning, (iv) mobility, (v) self-direction (vi) capacity for independent living, and (vii) economic sufficiency; and
> (e) reflects the person's need for a combination and sequence of special, interdisciplinary, or generic care, treatment, or other services which are of lifelong or extended duration and individually planned and coordinated.
>
> [42 USC 6102 (7)]

To help individuals cope with the effects of developmental disability on their ability to deal with the requirements of their daily functioning in society, service providers have recently tried to design educational, residential and health services that include individuals in the mainstream of society as much as possible. Thus, early intervention services for infants with developmental disability or developmental delay (Turnbull & Turnbull, 1990) and for their families have moved from specialist centre-based programs to generic family intervention programs designed to give children and their families access to needed support within generic services (Bailey & Simeonsson, 1988; Dunst, Trivette & Deal, 1988). Attempts to develop integrated or more inclusive services for students at the school level have already been alluded to, while schools themselves are being encouraged to prepare their students with developmental disabilities to take their place in non-institutional care environments through participation in well-designed transition education programs (Horner, Meyer & Fredericks, 1986; Wilcox & Bellamy, 1982). Finally, at the adult level, more normalised community-living arrangements are being encouraged than were provided by the earlier institutional care models, while governments are generally encouraging agencies to abandon the sheltered workshop model of providing work for adults, in favour of supported employment alternatives in regular workplace settings (Australian Government, 1987).

What, then, are the challenges posed by these policies of inclusion for people with developmental disabilities who are attempting to participate more fully in the normal experiences of twentieth-century living? Clearly, a comprehensive analysis of that question is beyond the scope of this book. It is very clear, however, that efforts are needed to improve the social, interactive or communicative relationships *among* those with developmental disabilities and *between* these people and their non-handicapped communicative partners, either at home, in schools, in recreational settings or in their workplaces.

To achieve these improvements, a great deal needs to be done to develop the *attitudes, knowledge* and *skills* of all of those who work with people with developmental disabilities and, indeed, of those increasing numbers of people in the wider community who will come in contact during their daily lives with people with developmental disabilities, including those with communication disabilities. While a traditionally held view may have been to focus on the individual with the disability in planning an educational intervention, as in learning a new skill to facilitate mainstreaming, a more fruitful, or at least complementary, view may be to intervene directly with those engaged in providing care, staff training, policy development, institutional research or related matters. In other words, there may be much to be gained from a reappraisal of the ways in which our society's educational and care-giving processes work to either facilitate or inhibit the development of interpersonal communication skills for those with developmental disabilities.

Theoretical Considerations

This book is an attempt to examine ways in which communication can be enhanced through interventions in naturalistic settings. It comprises the efforts of a number of professionals who set out to learn more about the ways in which communicative behaviour can be developed in clients of different ages who have developmental disabilities affecting communication. Each of the authors has set out to present an up-to-date review of relevant theory and research and then, in most cases, to design an investigation that attempts to address practitioner needs in working with clients with communication disabilities, in a contemporary educational or other human service setting.

Before introducing each of the studies reported in the following chapters, it may be appropriate to consider their common theoretical underpinnings. The view of communication learning that is implicit in the following chapters recognises the developments in recent theory. Earlier work in developing language-training programs for those with disabilities was based on attempts to introduce gradually more complex sentence structures, using principles of applied behaviour analysis (for example, Kent, 1974). More recently, Lois Bloom was credited with the "semantic revolution" in language development theory, by drawing attention to word classes — for example, object names and action words — which were observed in the developing language of young children (Bloom, 1970; Bloom & Lahey, 1978). Interestingly, children sometimes uttered the same word to refer to different word classes or relationships. Perhaps the best-known example is Bloom's description of her young daughter's use of the phrase "Mommy sock". This utterance was used on some occasions to refer to the sock owned by her mother while on others it referred to the act of putting on the sock (or perhaps was a request to do so) (Bloom, 1970, p 5).

A stronger contemporary interest in young children's development of language and communication skills can be found in the work dealing with pragmatics that was reported in the 1970s. An early report (1975) by Michael Halliday described the way his son used language to achieve social communicative purposes when he was between the ages of about 6 and 18 months. Thus, language can be used for such purposes as regulating the behaviour of others, obtaining services from people and for amusing oneself, among other purposes. The ways in which children develop the ability to convey particular ideas, or to intend particular effects (such as requesting services or eliciting humour) on their communicative partners, became of interest to researchers (Bates, 1976; Bates, Benigni, Bretherton, Camaioni & Volterra, 1977). This interest in pragmatics became important in providing a theoretical framework for students of language development in people with disabilities, as the following chapters will show.

Pragmatics appears to be a concept that is linked to the motivation or desire to communicate in a particular context (Bernstein & Tiegerman, 1992), and this appears to be critical for those with disabilities. It has been reported that many individuals have been exposed to language-training programs aimed at instilling a number of syntactic forms but could not use them later for purposes of social interaction when in a (different) setting that required the use of those trained forms (Garcia & deHaven, 1974; Tierney, 1981). Similarly, O'Connor and Hermelin reported as early as 1962 that mentally handicapped subjects observed in their research were unable to communicate or disinterested in communicating or using trained linguistic forms when given the opportunity to do so. It seems important, then, to invest time and energy in research that may uncover something of the circumstances leading to or, alternatively, exacerbating the unwillingness of many individuals with developmental disability to communicate, even with the help of those linguistic, manual or perhaps electronic means that are known or available to them.

While the shifts in focus of interest by language theorists and researchers can easily become very confusing to the newcomer with a general or an applied interest in this field, two publications of the late 1970s may be very helpful. Bloom and Lahey (1978) integrated the various directions in which language development theory had developed during the earlier phases to create a model that placed equal emphasis on *form*, *content* and *use*. "Form" referred to the speech or other communication mode used by the learner and also included the syntactic forms that emerge in a young speaker's early language. "Content" referred to the vocabulary or semantic features of a new speaker's emerging language as well as the semantic relationships within that language. "Use" referred to the communicative functions that language serves for the speaker and is subsumed by the concept of pragmatics discussed earlier. The interactive nature of the form, content and use aspects of early communicative behaviour is an important feature of language development, according to Bloom and Lahey, who see developments in each area as both facilitating, and being facilitated by, developments in the others.

A transactional approach to language development was described by McLean and Snyder-McLean (1978) and echoes many of the sentiments of the Bloom and Lahey model. What is especially interesting to the present discussion, however, is the sharp focus in the transactional model of the social interactive basis of language development. This focus turns our attention to the ways in which speakers use language to achieve social communicative purposes. A speaker's intentions in using communicative behaviour or in uttering particular words can become an important area of interest in trying to design intervention programs for people with delayed language development.

Authors of the chapters presented in the following pages have taken the "transactional" or social-communicative functional view of language development as they have set out to learn more about the communicative behaviour of particular age and ability groups of individuals involved in communicative behaviour. However, before introducing these chapters in broad outline, it is appropriate to define the terminology used in this book, with some clarification of the terms "communication", "language" and "speech". While slightly different definitions of these terms may be found in some chapters, the following definitions should provide a useful starting point for embarking on the remainder of this book.

It is clear that a useful notion of the term "communication" needs to take account of the interactive processes between speaker and listener. A limitation of earlier training with individuals having severe disorders of communication was the absence of the training effects in naturally occurring interactive settings. Communication should be seen, therefore, as a process for sharing ideas between people. "Communication" is a more general term than "speech" or "language", and it can take place, though perhaps crudely, outside of the conventional speech and language forms. According to McCormick and Schiefelbusch (1984, pp 4–5),

> The defining characteristic of communication is that it entails an exchange of ideas and intentions . . . It involves knowledge of social and cultural conventions such as conversational turn-taking, forms of address, standard verbal routines and sufficient motivation to apply this knowledge.

In considering the distinction between speech and language, Bloom and Lahey proposed that language can be defined differently for different purposes, according to which dimension of language is under consideration. Thus, a definition depends upon the context in which one asks the question "What is language?". So, in considering the learning of language and assisting that process in children with language development problems, Bloom and Lahey defined language as a "code whereby ideas about the world are represented through a conventional system of arbitrary signals for communication" (1978, p 4).

Compared to communication and language, speech is a much more restricted concept involved in the transmission of ideas and intents. Owens described speech as a "mode or verbal means of communicating" (1984, p 3) involving neuromuscular coordination for the particular combination of speech sounds (or phonemes) characteristic of a given language. McCormick and Schiefelbusch (1984) indicated that speech is only one of many vehicles used in the production of language. Gesturing, manual signing, writing and using pictures, diagrams, body postures and facial expressions are other modes that can be used for language. Thus, speech can be seen as a subset of language, itself a part of the wider process of communication.

An Outline of the Following Chapters

This chapter began with an anecdote concerning the apparent efficacy of regular class placement for some children with severe intellectual disability. According to senior teachers at that school, improvements in speech and language abilities were noticed shortly after the children's transfer from special classes to regular classes where they were integrated or mainstreamed with children of their own age.

The association between young children's development of language and of play skills has long been a topic of interest to observers of child development. Drawing upon a number of standardised assessment approaches, Nancy Butterfield has used work pioneered by Westby (1980) in assessing the development of language and of play skills in a small group of young children with severe intellectual disability. The ability to let certain objects stand for, or represent, other objects is called symbolisation, and she identifies this ability, which emerges from children's experiences in developing play skills, as an important stage in the acquisition of language. Her investigation, reported in Chapter 2, points to an association between children's play and language skills, as demonstrated by the assessments that were carried out. That association points to the possibility of differential intervention needs related to individual children's play skills, and the implications for practitioners are discussed.

Chapter 3 takes the issue of the effects of the classroom setting on communication a little further by reporting on an investigation of children with mild intellectual disability attending regular preschool classes. In that chapter, Diana Messervy shows how the language and other forms of communicative behaviour used by the children when requesting a desired object (a toy in this case) were influenced by various factors in the setting. In particular, she identifies the different forms of communication used by the children to make requests and the influence on these behaviours of the size of the group in which the child was a member and of the children's developmental levels. A discussion then follows, which presents the implications of these findings for preschool teaching practices, along with some suggested strategies for promoting requesting behaviour in this population of language-delayed preschool children.

A different focus is presented by Kathleen Dice in Chapter 4. Here, attention is turned to teaching students with communication impairment to augment their communicative behaviour with a manual-signing system. The difficult question of deciding upon the detail of the vocabulary content used in an initial signing program is addressed very comprehensively. Competing sources of vocabulary content include knowledge of the child's language acquisition, consideration of the child's functional communication needs in particular environments and, significantly, an appreciation of the physical constraints on learning to perform particular manual signs. These issues are reviewed in a discussion that draws very widely on research in this area.

Returning to the matter of setting or contextual influences on communicative behaviour, Ken Linfoot presents in Chapter 5 a report on an investigation in which the communicative behaviour of a group of school students with severe and profound intellectual disability was studied over a 12-month period. This study showed how pragmatic features of the children's verbal and non-verbal communicative behaviour varied according to the type of lesson presented by the teacher. Effects associated with the developmental levels of the students were also observed. The report contains a number of implications for teachers and caregivers who work with children from this population and who need strategies to enhance their communicative behaviour. Indeed, the conclusion that what is achieved in so-called language lessons may not be as useful as the language learning in less formal situations may come as something of a surprise. Nevertheless, these findings appear consistent with the theory base used for much of the work reported in this book.

Sue Healy's report in Chapter 6 provides some encouragement for readers whose interest is in enhancing communicative behaviour in people with multiple impairments who are, as a result, unable to use verbal language forms. This single-case study examines the effects on the adolescent school student's initiations of and responses to communication after his introduction to an electronic communication aid that produces synthetic speech. Although highly specific in its area of investigation and in its methodology, this study has demonstrated that a student with multiple disabilities is able to communicate with this particular piece of technology and is not overwhelmed by its complexity or restricted to using it on demand as a "party trick".

The studies presented in Chapters 2 to 6 explore, across a wide range of ages of people with developmental disabilities, various attempts to implement strategies to enhance the communicative behaviour of this population. What links the various approaches is a concern to place the teaching of communicative behaviour in environments that are functional for the individuals concerned. Moreover, the approaches generally place at least equal emphasis on helping individuals to increase their range of the pragmatic functions of communication, or of the communicative intents at their disposal. Considerable caution should be exercised, of course, in the interpretation of and generalisation from findings obtained from research studies such as these. The studies were conducted using small samples, in most cases in only one location; there was often an absence of control groups (though some studies used designs where subjects were able to serve as their own controls); and research subjects were rarely chosen randomly but were identified as being available and cooperative with the research effort.

Each of the authors has indicated the particular restrictions on the external validity of the specific study. Nevertheless, it is suggested that each study may offer practitioners some insights into teaching methods that may be useful in settings akin to those reported here. Moreover, the aggregation of these findings with others reported elsewhere may contribute to that bank of research data that will help to show the way toward practices that may be more generally useful.

In Chapter 7, Michael Arthur does attempt to point the way toward issues and themes that are relevant to the theory and practice of communication training into the foreseeable future. One theme is the concern that the vocalisations and gestures that have traditionally been interpreted as non-communicative, or indeed aberrant in some individuals with severe intellectual disabilities, may be communicative after all. Ways in which teachers and caregivers may be assisted to recognise these and develop more appropriate communicative forms thus become important research and training tasks. Further, the commitment of school systems and community services to provide the necessary support for individuals with communication disability and their caregivers in normalised community settings remains an important challenge, in the light of our current beliefs in the efficacy of naturalistic intervention settings where there is adequate specialist support for caregivers. These and other issues are canvassed in this chapter, along with a survey of recent research directions in this exciting contemporary field of study.

The final chapter is an attempt by three of the contributors to draw together an account of how the findings of recent research in this field can be used to influence practical intervention for people with communication disorders. The discussion focuses on using naturalistic environments in everyday home, childcare, educational, residential or work settings. Intervention methods are based on facilitating social interaction skills rather than using a didactic instructional approach. As a result, it is clear that a wide variety of people need to learn some basic skills in order to enhance the opportunities for this population to learn and use communication behaviour. The strategies described in Chapter 8 should help people working with or caring for this population to develop those skills.

This chapter has attempted to explain the theoretical basis of language and communication development underpinning much of the contemporary work in this field. In particular, our understanding of the ways in which social interaction processes may be disrupted for people with intellectual disabilities has been helped considerably by this theoretical structure. Perhaps more importantly, the transactional model of communication and language development has been helpful in the design of intervention studies to assist individuals with communication problems. It is hoped that the studies and techniques reported in this book may be of assistance to other practitioners and caregivers in this important and rewarding area of human services.

References

Australian Government (1987). Disability services program, general information on eligible services. Competitive employment training and placement services. Notes from the Australian Department of Community Services and Health.

Bailey, D.B. & Simeonsson, R.J. (1988). *Family assessment in early intervention*. Columbus: Charles E. Merrill.

Bates, E. (1976). *Language and context: The acquisition of pragmatics*. New York: Academic Press.

Bates, E., Benigni, L., Bretherton, I., Camaioni, L. & Volterra, V. (1977). From gesture to the first word: On cognitive and social prerequisites. In M. Lewis & L.A. Rosenblum (eds), *Interaction, conversation and the development of language*. New York: John Wiley & Sons.

Bernstein, D.K. & Tiegerman, E. (1992). *Language and communication disorders in children*, 3rd Edition. Columbus: Charles E. Merrill.

Bloom, L. (1970). *Language development: Form and function in emerging grammars*. Cambridge: MIT Press.

Bloom, L. & Lahey, M. (1978). *Language development and language disorders*. New York: John Wiley & Sons.

Dunst, C.J., Trivette, C. & Deal, A. (1988). *Enabling and empowering families: Principles and guidelines for practice*. Cambridge: Brookline Books.

Garcia, E.E. & deHaven, E.D. (1974). Use of operant techniques in the establishment and generalization of language: A review and analysis. *American Journal of Mental Deficiency 79*, 169–78.

Horner, R.H., Meyer, L.M. & Fredericks, H.D. (eds) (1986). *Education of learners with severe handicaps: Exemplary service strategies*. Baltimore: Paul H. Brookes.

Kent, L. (1974). *Language acquisition program for the severely retarded*. Champaign: Research Press.

McCormick, L. & Schiefelbusch, R.L. (eds) (1984). *Early language intervention*. Columbus: Charles E. Merrill.

McDonnell, J., Wilcox, B. & Hardman, M. (1991). *Secondary programs for students with developmental disability*. Boston: Allyn & Bacon.

McLean, J.E. & Snyder-McLean, L.K. (1978). *A transactional approach to early language training*. Columbus: Charles E. Merrill.

Nirje, B. (1970). The normalization principle: Implications and comments. *British Journal of Mental Subnormality 16*, 62–70.

O'Connor, N. & Hermelin, B. (1962). *Speech and thought in severe subnormality: An experimental study*. Oxford: Pergamon Press.

Owens, R.E. (1984). *Language development: An introduction*. Columbus: Charles E. Merrill.

Tierney, I. (1981). Behaviour modification in communication deficit. In W.I. Frazer & R. Grieve (eds), *Communicating with normal and retarded children*. Bristol: John Wright & Sons.

Turnbull, A.P. & Turnbull, H.R. (1990). *Families, professionals and exceptionality: A special partnership*, 2nd Edition. Columbus: Charles E. Merrill.

Westby, C.E. (1980). Assessment of language and cognitive abilities through play. *Language, Speech and Hearing Services in Schools 11*, 154–68.

Wilcox, B. & Bellamy, G.T. (1982). *Design of high school programs for severely handicapped students*. Baltimore: Paul H. Brookes.

Wolfensberger, W. (1972). *The principle of normalization in human services*. Toronto: National Institute on Mental Retardation.

Chapter 2

Play as an Assessment and Intervention Strategy for Children with Language and Intellectual Disabilities

Nancy Butterfield

Charles Sturt University-Mitchell
Bathurst, NSW

This chapter explores young children's development of the ability to symbolise and particularly the role of this ability in the development of both play and language. Similarities in the development of language and play were reported in the work of Sinclair (1973), Fein (1975), Lowe (1975) and Leibergott and Swope (1976). Later studies reflect continuing interest in this area (Westby, 1980; McCune-Nicholich & Carol, 1981; Corrigan, 1982; Ungerer & Sigman, 1984; Atlas & Lapidus, 1988; Beeghly, Weiss-Perry & Cicchetti, 1989; Kennedy, Sheridan, Radlinski & Beeghly, 1991).

The study reported here investigated the development of symbolisation in the play and language of young children with an intellectual disability, and found that this skill provides a relevant basis for assessing stages in language development in order to provide a relevant basis for therapy. However, in situations where the difference between mental age and chronological age is great and the student is at an age where play is no longer appropriate, it becomes more relevant to base assessment and therapy on age-appropriate leisure activities, together with observations of interpersonal interactions throughout daily living routines.

The theoretical base for this study stems from the work of Piaget (1962), who saw symbolic ability as an indication of underlying cognitive development. Both play and language can provide outward measures of this symbolic ability. While language is measured by outward signs of communication, both verbal and nonverbal, and provides a measure of social symbolic ability, play is measured by signs of pretending and provides a measure of personal symbolic ability.

The literature relating to the representational nature of language and the development of the ability to symbolise reveals a developmental progression in both play and language. Parallel stages in development appear to reflect an underlying common base. McCune-Nicholich and Carol (1981) hypothesise that "... an underlying cognitive development renders the child capable of the hierarchical symbolic combinations observed in both play and language" (p 8) and propose a developmental interdependence between the two.

The role of symbol use in language is also discussed by Bloom and Lahey (1978), who define language as "... a code whereby ideas about the world are presented through a conventional system of arbitrary signals for communication" (p 4). Thus language is a means of representing knowledge of objects, events or relationships and is based on a referential or representational system that uses symbols, generally words, to stand for objects, people and events. Knowledge of the world provides the basis for the content of language (meaning); the means of representing that knowledge in a linguistic code forms the structure of language (form); and the ability to use that structure to gain different ends in differing circumstances provides the functional aspect of language (use). "Language consists of some aspect of content or meaning that is coded or represented by linguistic form for some purpose or use in a particular context" (Bloom & Lahey, 1978, p 11).

Communication is essentially, therefore, a social phenomenon and refers to the signalling behaviour in an interaction between two or more persons, where shared understanding is created (Warren & Kaiser, 1988). It involves initiation and response in a two-way process of making one's intentions known and understanding the intentions of others. Language systems provide the means for communication to occur, where the code used is recognised by the culture of the individual. The code may be in the form of words, gestures, facial expressions, formal signing systems or pictorial symbols that act to signal the communicative intent of the interaction. Where a spoken code cannot be used, alternative symbolic systems can be taught as a means to augment existing vocal abilities.

Play is the dominant developmental activity in the growth of communication skills in young children. Fewell and Kaminski (1988) describe play as an activity that is intrinsically motivating for the child. In addition, play is essentially a spontaneous, voluntary and self-generated activity which involves enjoyment and also provides the social basis for language development.

Discussion in this chapter will cover the following topics:

1. The development of representational ability
2. Cognitive prerequisites for language development
3. Social aspects of language development
4. Parallels in the development of play and language
5. Implications for intervention
6. Report of a small-scale study assessing language and play abilities
7. Implications for classroom practices
8. Conclusions.

The Development of Representational Ability

Piaget's model of cognitive development for normal children provides a description of the stages from birth, where development in the first two years (the sensorimotor period) provides the foundation for further development. This foundation is not a quantitative accumulation of ideas and facts but rather is seen as a qualitative change in the processes of thought and the acquisition of concepts, so that gradually the child's view of reality is changed from an egocentric view to one recognising the reality of others (McCormick & Schiefelbusch, 1984).

Piaget did not describe a model of language development but placed language as one form of representational ability or symbolic function (Owens, 1984). The capacity for mental representation emerges during the sixth and final stages of the sensorimotor period of development. The emergence of symbolic play in the sensorimotor period is seen as important to the development of further mental representational ability.

Symbolic activity is characterised by the substitution of one or more objects for the object that would usually be involved in the activity. The child also shows awareness of that substitution by signs of pleasure or lack of seriousness (Bates, 1979). In symbolic play the child represents objects and events with substitutes or copies, and imitative actions become internalised. For example, a relationship between an absent object (cup) and a symbolic object (leaf) is expressed when the child uses the leaf as a cup in play. Language can also be seen to require similar representational ability. Just as the object used in play indicates that the child is aware that it is a representation of the real object, so too does the use of a word indicate that the word is not the object but only a representation of that object (Westby, 1980).

The ability to form representations develops gradually as the child interacts with the environment. In the first month the child shows no sign of intentional play behaviour. As the child begins to produce simple reactions that provide pleasure, these are repeated with familiar objects. When adaptive play begins, the child uses a similar object as a substitute for another. This develops into symbolic play, when any object can be used to signify another. For symbolic enactment, the objects normally used need not be present (Dunst, 1980).

Symbolic activity is seen as being communicative when language is the medium and private when play is the medium (Bates, 1979). The early representational ability that the child develops in the sensorimotor period is private and highly individual. Consider, for example, imagination, imagery, symbolic play, dreaming and drawing. The use of language as a socially communicable form of symbolic behaviour can free the child from his or her own world of present objects and allow for further development. This is significant in that representational ability continues to progress in the following cognitive stages with the use of language as a symbolic function.

The use of language as the symbolic means to represent reality requires greater abstraction than play. In play, the symboliser (an object standing for or representing another) can be similar or linked in some way to the object being represented. However, in language, words do not resemble the form or function of the real object, and their meaning may depend on the relationships expressed in the grammatical structures of the statement. There is an increasing dependency on the maturing levels of symbolic ability for the child to become a competent user of language (Westby, 1980).

It is believed that the ability to demonstrate double knowledge — that is, symbolic function — has considerable significance for the development of the ability to use words in language and that, in fact, a child who lacks the development of symbolic representation will also lack the ability to develop any language system as one form of representation (Morehead & Morehead, 1974). McHale, Simeonsson, Marcus and Olley (1980) examined the developmental status of communicative behaviours in relation to symbolic play in eleven autistic children and found "children's symbolic language usage was highly correlated with their symbolic functioning in other domains (i.e. symbolic play)" (p 309).

Language and pretend play both require that a child mentally represents reality. What is important is the means by which children learn to represent ideas and concepts. Representation is an outcome of the sensorimotor period, where directly acting on objects in play enables the child to recognise similarities between objects, which forms the beginning of representational intelligence.

Cognitive Prerequisites for Language Development

Interest in better understanding the cognitive prerequisites for language is evident in the work of Bloom (1970), Bricker and Bricker (1974), Halliday (1975), Bowerman (1978) and Bruner (1983), who were interested in how meaning is conveyed in language, which is a form of symbolic ability used to represent cognitive thought. Their work described the course of development of children's utterances and contrasted with an earlier preoccupation with the development of syntax.

Their research led the way to the realisation that it is how children learn to represent ideas and concepts that is important. Bruner (1983) stressed that play teaches the child the effects created within the environment by his or her behaviour and helps integrate what the child has learnt about objects and people. The child eventually uses words for the purpose of further learning, instead of actions as in early play, and is more effectively able to satisfy needs and to control and interact with others.

Bricker and Bricker (1974) developed an approach that considered both the child's sensorimotor intelligence and prelinguistic development. They were interested in the use of imitation as a basis for training and the use of motoric cues or actions together with sounds to represent objects (performatives) in order to bridge the verbal gap. As they explained, ". . . for the young child an object is what it does, or what he can do with it. The child's development from inactive knowledge to symbolic knowledge about the world emerges through his direct interaction and action on the environment" (p 453).

This view of early cognitive development has been significant in influencing approaches to language intervention for people with intellectual disabilities (Kangas & Lloyd, 1988). However, great caution is necessary in considering the significance of cognitive prerequisites as a basis for the development of symbolic communication, as the relationship between cognition and language development is quite complex. Rice (1983) described six models that have been developed to explain this relationship. The proposal that cognition ". . . is necessary but not sufficient for language acquisition" (Kangas & Lloyd, 1988) has had its greatest influence on language programs for students with severe intellectual disabilities. This view claims that a cognitive base is necessary for language to develop but will not ensure language development as linguistic factors are also necessary. For example, Bates, Camaioni and Volterra (1975) reported that the ability to use preverbal, intentional communication corresponds with Piaget's sensorimotor stage 5 abilities, and the ability to use words corresponds to sensorimotor stage 6. Both cognitive and linguistic abilities need to be considered.

Kangas and Lloyd (1988), after reviewing several studies linking cognition and language, cautioned that conclusions have been based on data showing a correlation between cognitive development and language measures but not proving a cause and effect relationship. Given this evidence, the complexity of the relationship and the number of possible models proposed, it appears that there is a relationship between cognition and language in which each supports and facilitates growth in the other (Rice & Kemper, 1984). As a result, it seems necessary to consider both cognitive and language abilities rather than to target one in isolation or wait for predetermined cognitive prerequisites.

There have also been attempts to link specific sensorimotor attainments to the development of language. The ability to imitate, understanding causality and object permanence, means-end abilities, and the abilities involved in spatial relations and symbolic play may be measured to indicate a child's cognitive readiness for language development (Dunst, 1980).

Relating to objects and understanding object permanence have been described as functional abilities necessary for the inclusion of content in language or for acquiring and organising experiences so that the child can talk about them. Means-end abilities and an understanding of operational causality have been described as being related to the ability to use language as a communicative strategy to achieve a desired end. Finally, imitation is seen to be relevant to the development of language form and corresponds with the use of conventional linguistic modes (McCormick & Schiefelbusch, 1984).

Reichle and Karlan (1985) argued that there is lack of empirical support for claims that specific cognitive abilities are prerequisites for language development. In addition, Ungerer and Sigman (1984) reported little relationship between specific sensorimotor behaviours and language skills. Westby (1980) indicated that it is not necessary to posit a causal relationship between specific language skills and specific cognitive abilities. Instead, it is more important to recognise that ". . . some cognitive abilities consistently precede or occur with certain communicative intentions and linguistic structures" (p 154). Such cognitive abilities are developed at the same time as communicative and language skills, in play and social interactive settings (McCormick & Shane, 1984; Rice, 1986).

The assessment of cognitive attainments of young children with intellectual disabilities can be difficult. Due to the varied nature of each individual's disabilities, the development of individual components of sensorimotor skill is not uniform within individuals or within the population (Rogers, 1977; Snyder-McLean, McLean & Etter, 1988). Rogers assessed the sensorimotor skills of 40 profoundly retarded institutionalised children, aged from eight to fourteen, and found that attainments followed the same sequence as typical children's development, but performance across the various domains was not equal for individuals.

Kangas and Lloyd (1988, p 213) concluded that "... there is no clear evidence that language rests on any well specified cognitive prerequisite skills ... Although it can be readily agreed that there must be some relationship between cognition and language, it should be recognised that the nature of this relationship is not clearly understood."

Language is seen to build its structures on cognitive capacities, resulting in a developmental dependence such that one system requires input from the other. The cognitive capacities permit language to occur, but they do not cause language development (Bates, 1979). It is the interdependence between linguistic and non-linguistic factors that occurs during the emergence of symbolic capacity that is significant.

Social Aspects of Language Development

A further important aspect of language development that is related to the cognitive-based theory is the social functions of language — the fact that children intend to communicate certain meanings through their actions and utterances. Bowerman (1978), Halliday (1975), Bates (1979) and Bruner (1983) all show interest in the role of the context of the utterance to examine the function or communicative intent of children's language.

Bruner was particularly interested in the nature of early social interactions between child and caregiver as a critical element in promoting the development of meaning in communication. Play and games provide the ideal support for language acquisition, emphasising both the cognitive and social aspects of early language acquisition. Play teaches the child the effects created within the environment by his or her behaviour, and integrates what the child has learnt about objects and people. The first games played by child and caretaker, such as peek-a-boo, are significant in that they are based on language and their existence depends on language. In addition, they assign turn-taking roles and shared attention to an ordered sequence. In fact, "... play measures may bear an especially strong correlation with language skills because they index social awareness ..." (Ungerer & Sigman, 1984, in Mundy, Sigman, Ungerer & Sherman, 1987, p 350).

Early social interactions take place as the child develops during the early sensorimotor stages. Infants are seen as progressively developing goal-directed activity (Bates, 1979). In the first instance, a child will reach to obtain a desired object. It is not until there is an understanding that adults can be used to help obtain that object, that the child is able to communicate intentionally with others (Sugarman, 1984). Development of the social aspect of communication has begun.

Bates et al. (1975), Halliday (1975), Bloom and Lahey (1978), Sugarman (1984) and Dunst and Lowe (1986) all propose a developmental progression in the social abilities of infants between birth and two years as they increasingly display intentional communication with others. Early acts serve to satisfy material needs or maintain social interactions, and their outcomes are progressively predictable. As a result, the child develops the ability to use gestures and vocalisations purposefully to indicate desired ends. Such prelinguistic acts develop from idiosyncratic communicative behaviours which gradually approximate more standardised forms, until the child can use words and language with the same intent as those early acts had.

Halliday (1975) described how a non-disabled child systematically develops a series of communicative functions, each expressing a different type of social interaction and behaviour which is directed toward achieving particular regulatory or instrumental control (or pragmatic function) with a communicative partner.

The examination of the social basis for language development has therefore resulted in an expansion of the view that language is a structurally based system alone. However, important developments have highlighted the interdependence of the meaning (content) conveyed by language, the function intended (use) and the means (form) used to express these. Language, in fact, cannot be viewed without attention to all three aspects: form, content and use (Bloom & Lahey, 1978).

Parallels in the Development of Play and Language

Interest in the development of representational abilities and the ability to symbolise has led to research investigating the relationships between the development of language and play. Early studies described stages in play that can be identified while children are learning language. Fein (1975) reported that in symbolic play, the child at first chooses a symboliser similar to the object being represented and later selects less-related objects. Lowe (1975) found that children practised acts in self-related play before transferring these to doll-related play, the latter corresponding to the time when children started putting words together. Leibergott and Swope (1976) investigated the development of symbolic schemes in the pre-operational period (following the sensorimotor period) to identify ways in which stages in play could provide a basis for language therapy. McCune-Nicholich and

Carol (1981) and Westby (1980) investigated the development of sequences for both play and language. It was found that children progressed through a sequence of play levels but at varying rates, and that parallel stages in language could be mapped.

There has been continued interest in examining the systematic relationships found to occur between play and language in normally developing infants (Corrigan, 1982; Ungerer & Sigman, 1984), in young children with developmental delays (Beeghly et al, 1989; Kennedy et al, 1991) and in children with severe pervasive developmental disorders (Atlas & Lapidus, 1988; McHale et al, 1980).

Beeghly et al (1989) found that, while children with Down syndrome showed delays in learning to play, the overall developmental trends in cognitive functioning and play maturity were similar to those of normally developing infants. On the other hand, Kennedy et al (1991) examined six children with a range of developmental delays in a longitudinal study and found interesting variations highlighting the irregularities in patterns of development in such populations. Their study also demonstrated the importance of play as an assessment and intervention strategy for such groups of young children.

Observing play sequences reveals a progression in the development of symbolic abilities as shown by the increasing complexity of pretend play. Pretending is evident if the child performs everyday activities in the absence of necessary materials, substitutes one object for another, performs activities usually associated with another person, treats inanimate objects as animate, does not carry activities to their usual outcome or displays an awareness of the nonliteral quality of the activity (McCune-Nicholich & Carol, 1981).

In the first instance of symbolic ability, the child performs usual movements in the presence of an appropriate object. For example, on seeing a pillow the child lies on it as if to sleep. Later a doll will be put to sleep, indicating projection of the symbolic behaviour to other persons and objects. After such simple schemes develop, the child will apply them to various actors or objects and, later, will also include a sequence of related events. As the child begins to substitute one object for another, objects with similar features are first sought. Play also begins to contain planned elements, such as announcing the game and searching for objects, so that eventually pretend activities can be planned and mentally represented in advance, with words being used to assist in this.

At the same time, progression in the ability to involve others in play is also developing. Initial play is described as exploratory, where the infant investigates, explores and tests through object manipulation. Independent or solitary play follows where the child uses appropriate play actions with objects, but plays without reference to others. In parallel play, the child continues to play alone but in close physical proximity to peers with similar materials. At the associative stage, the play appears to be organised around a common activity, with a limited number of approaches and responses to peers evident. This becomes cooperative play when the child regularly approaches and responds to peers and adults. Finally, symbolic play enables deliberate misrepresentation of reality using pretend or miniature props (Musselwhite, 1986). Play stages can be seen to provide an index for social awareness.

A decreasing dependence on contextual support and an increasing ability to use words for the symbolic function are evident in the acquisition of communication and language skills. The early stages of communicative intent have been described as developing from acts based on physical and affective needs, with preverbal abilities such as gestures and vocalisations being significant precursors to later verbal abilities (Bates et al, 1975). First word forms emphasise performative functions and later take on semantic roles but remain dependent on the context for meaning. With the development of increasing symbolic ability, relationships can be expressed in two-word utterances and words can be used to represent objects and people not present.

There are two possible features that influence the discussion of parallel stages in language and play development. First, both are symbolic systems that are sequenced according to rules in order to represent events. Secondly, both symbolic systems are used in a social context for the purpose of social interaction (Ungerer & Sigman, 1984). Examination of play sequences shows growing maturity in both symbol systems and social abilities. At the same time, language development shows increasing maturity in the use of symbols and in the ability to use those symbols to interact with others. Language and play both share a social and communicative function.

Parallel development in pretend play and language usage has been mapped, with both domains sharing the underlying cognitive attainment of symbolic ability. Given that play is a medium that enables symbolic ability to be observed, it provides a context for the assessment of and intervention in language development. Play sessions are child-centred and allow the child to be spontaneous in demonstrating communication abilities. Following assessment, intervention sessions based on play can begin with the skills and interests of the child, maintaining the essential features of both the cognitive and social bases for language development.

Of particular interest in this regard is the Symbolic Play Scale Checklist developed by Westby (1980). In this checklist, ten stages of play and language are described, covering an age span ranging from nine to twelve months to five years. At each stage of play there is a parallel stage of language development. The play sequence reflects a progression in the development of symbolic abilities as shown by the increasing complexity of pretend play. The language sequence shows progressions from communicative intent, semantic concepts and syntactic structures.

The Westby scale was developed from a Piaget-based language program used with children with severe and moderate intellectual disabilities in special education classes. When the developmental patterns of normal children were compared with those of the children with intellectual disabilities, Westby found that both groups followed the same sequences in play and language stages. Later studies support this finding. Ungerer and Sigman (1984) found the consistent relationship between play and language to be due to the ability to translate experiences into symbols. Mundy et al (1987) found that play variables correlated with language development, and that nonverbal communication correlated with language development, but that play and nonverbal communication variables were not correlated. Kennedy et al (1991) reported a longitudinal study where they found correspondence between language development and symbolic play in six children with developmental delays.

These studies support the findings of parallel progressions in play and language and their application to populations with developmental delay. The implications for intervention are now examined as the assessment of play variables relative to language abilities can provide important information for remediation (Westby, 1980).

Implications for Intervention

The developments in theory and research reported earlier have led to a renewed interest in the means to assess language abilities and to provide intervention for language-delayed children.

In relation to assessment procedures, Fewell and Kaminski (1988) indicated that play provides a more valid indication of the child's actual functioning level than more formal assessment procedures.

> Because observation of play is an unobtrusive and nonthreatening procedure, children will more likely behave in a more typical manner than when asked to follow an unfamiliar adult's directions in a testing situation. In addition, responding to standardized test items may be impossible for some children with handicaps. (p 145)

More formal assessments may not provide accurate information regarding the child's abilities because of the unnatural environment in which they are administered, the bias that may exist against cultural or disability types, and the lack of functional information relevant to the application of skills being assessed (Linder, 1990).

Play-based assessment, on the other hand, can be carried out in an environment familiar to the child, with greater flexibility in equipment and conditions possible in order to overcome situations of bias due to a particular disability. A holistic view of the child is provided rather than a series of possibly fragmented reports from individual and unrelated assessments (Linder, 1990).

Play enables the interrelationship of cognitive, social and language development to be maintained through a unified approach (Linder, 1990). Importance is placed on the social context of learning, the environmental interactions that support that learning and recognition of the child's developing understanding of the world around him. Assessment and training procedures need to focus on the child, the caregiver and the quality of interactions across all daily environments (Dunst & Lowe, 1986; Siegel-Causey & Guess, 1989).

The traditional way of teaching language-delayed children by showing them labels for objects in clinical settings does not represent the way normal children creatively develop the means of using language as a symbolic system. In fact, children do not learn labels first but build on an accumulated understanding of communication for a variety of purposes prior to labelling objects. Bruner (1983) emphasised the need for play and games to provide support for cognitive and language development. Therapy could be designed around naturalistic interactions like those found to facilitate development in normal children. Language interventionists have begun to look to play and the development of representational ability as a means of structuring approaches to improve language development (Fewell & Kaminski, 1988; McCune-Nicholich & Carol, 1981; Westby, 1980).

Specific strategies to enhance the development of communicative abilities in natural settings have been described in the literature. For example, Dunst and Lowe (1986), Harrison, Lombardino and Stapell (1987) and Siegel-Causey and Guess (1989) proposed strategies to enhance communicative interactions for students with severe intellectual disabilities, functioning within the range of sensorimotor development. The focus in these approaches is on the recognition of non-symbolic means of communication (such as gestures and vocalisations) and on the enhancement of the quality of social interactions.

Scaffolding for cognitive schemes is a strategy that helps the child develop the ability to manipulate objects and so enhances the child's play activities. By demonstrating slightly more advanced object manipulation each time, the adult can encourage the child to engage in increasingly more complex play (Harrison et al, 1987).

Contingent responding is a necessary component when fostering increased social interactions. The fact that an adult responds predictably to the child's behaviours is important to the development of an association between a behaviour from one and the response from another (Dunst & Lowe, 1986; Siegel-Causey & Guess, 1989).

Activities that encourage *turn-taking* help to establish the reciprocal nature of give-and-take interactions at both the nonverbal and verbal levels. Playful, ritualised games provide opportunities for the child to practise interactional turns. It is possible to pause in such activities and signal to the child that a response is required for the game to continue (Harrison et al, 1987; Siegel-Causey & Guess, 1989).

Referencing refers to the situation where the adult directs the child's attention to an object that is required and then to the person who can be instrumental in obtaining that object for them. From this the understanding of the social aspect of communication is gained (Harrison et al, 1987).

Scaffolding for communication refers to a strategy that enables the child's present skills to be extended to the next level. By imitating the child's vocalisations or gestures and then modelling skills slightly in advance of these, the adult not only increases the interaction time but also encourages the child to elaborate on existing skills (Harrison et al, 1987; Siegel-Causey & Guess, 1989).

The above strategies are recommended for students functioning at the very early stages of cognitive and communicative development because of their power to increase student responsiveness in the social setting and at the same time to enhance their partners' ability to read behaviours and respond as if they are communicative (Butterfield, Arthur & Linfoot, 1992).

Halle (1984), Warren and Rogers-Warren (1985), McLean and Snyder-McLean (1987) recommend incidental teaching, delay procedures, the mand-model technique and an integration of these strategies for enhancing communication development in natural contexts and providing opportunities to introduce more formal systems of communication such as speech and/or signing and pictures.

Incidental teaching, a procedure originally described by Hart and Risley (1968), refers to the process whereby the caregiver takes advantage of situations that arise naturally out of unstructured settings. Play provides an ideal means to implement incidental strategies. For example, if the child indicates a desire for an object, the adult then uses this to encourage communication, providing clues and prompts if necessary. This procedure depends on child-initiated interactions and has been reported to be effective for extending verbal behaviours (Halle, 1984).

The mand-model technique, originally developed by Rogers-Warren and Warren (1980), provides the opportunity to develop the child's initial responding skills while teaching in the natural environment. The caregiver requests a response and then provides a model to teach the required response. This approach is dependent on the adult setting the interactive environment (such as providing toys for play), indicating that a response is required (such as a request for a toy) and modelling that response if necessary. Halle (1984) reports successful increases in verbalisations using this technique but cautions that it can become very adult-initiated and adult-centred, thus inhibiting the student's own initiation of responses. It does, however, appear to increase the quality of the interactions provided by caregivers.

Delay procedures (Halle, Marshall & Spradlin, 1979) provide a further natural-environment setting for intervention, where students are provided with increased opportunity to respond to cues other than adult verbalisations. The focus of this strategy is on initiating communication, whereas the previous strategies emphasised responding behaviours. Everyday or play situations provide many opportunities for adults to delay what is usually a predetermined routine.

Milieu teaching allows the benefits of each of these strategies to be integrated. The mand-model technique provides the control to enable effective increases in the rate of responses and structured training to occur in natural settings. This may be necessary in the early stages of the process. Delay procedures can be used when natural opportunities occur for the student to initiate communicative interactions. Incidental teaching can then be employed to improve the quality of communication once the student is effectively initiating communicative behaviours.

Each procedure can be used as a strategy involving play, pitched at the language and play abilities of the student. The essential features of these strategies include improving the quality of social interactions between the child and caregiver and maintaining the natural context as the learning environment (McLean & Snyder-McLean, 1987; Siegel-Causey & Guess, 1989). With play as a basis, language intervention using these strategies addresses both the cognitive and social aspects of development.

Intervention strategies, therefore, have been influenced by the shift away from focusing on the structure of language and toward an examination of the overall development that occurs in the early years. This stresses the recognition of the level of communicative and language abilities exhibited by the student. Early communicative attempts are fostered and encouraged so that they can be gradually extended to include the communication of intent through gestures, vocalisations and, finally, words. If the use of words does not develop according to the sequence of normal language development, then alternative or augmentative symbolic forms such as signing, pictorial symbols or natural gestures may need to be taught.

In addition, importance is placed on naturalistic interactions with specific strategies that can be used to enhance the social basis of communication development. For normally developing infants, play and social interactions in unstructured settings maintain the consistent growth and development of communicative abilities. For children with intellectual disabilities, specific attention needs to be given to stimulus materials and settings to enhance and maintain such interactions.

Report of a Small-scale Study Assessing Language and Play Abilities

The study involved six children with severe intellectual disabilities, who manifest a wide variety of individual differences and who were enrolled in one class in a special school. The children ranged in age from four to nine years, the average age being eight years. The varying nature of the children's disabilities made it imperative that each child be considered as an individual and not as part of a homogeneous group.

In view of the relationship between language and imaginative play, as manifestations of the same underlying symbolic function, it was hypothesised that school-aged children with severe intellectual disabilities and severe language delay will also show developmental delays in imaginative play. An implication of this is that learning about the levels of symbolic functioning in individual children may also be useful in designing strategies for language development in these children. The study was therefore designed to collect information on the language abilities and imaginative play skills of the target children.

Language assessment included all forms of communication manifested by each child, including gestures, signs, vocalisations and words. Assessment of play skills focused on the nature of the child's symbolic play, imaginative play and display of representational ability. If play and language do show parallels in development as discussed previously, then a relationship should be found between the language and play abilities of these children.

Instruments

The Symbolic Play Scale (Westby, 1980) was used to provide information for the assessment of language and play. In order to see if the results on the Westby Scale were consistent with levels of ability for language and symbolic usage, an independent assessment of these skills was also needed. The administration of the REEL Scale (Bzoch

& League, 1978) provided an independent measure of language. This instrument was devised to assess emergent language skills in infancy and to help in the early identification of young children who may have specific handicaps requiring early intervention. The scale is based on language ability levels found in a sample of infants from enriched environments, and consists of a series of age intervals with three items per interval for expressive and receptive language. The Uzgiris and Hunt Scales of Infant Psychological Development (Dunst, 1980) was used to measure sensorimotor development, as the ability to symbolise is an outcome of sensorimotor development. The scale measures specific abilities such as visual pursuit and awareness of the permanence of objects, means for obtaining desired environmental events, vocal and gestural imitation, operational causality, construction of objects in space and schemes for relating to objects. In this study, particular reference was made to the development of schemes for relating to objects as a measure of development in play.

Method

Language and play were observed in natural interaction situations within the classroom and were recorded in anecdotal notes made at the time. Tape-recording provided a means to later analyse language samples. Observations focused on individual children, although others may have been in the room or involved in the activities at the same time. Observations also included natural daily situations, such as meal times and change times, in order to gain an overall measure of communicative intent.

Play situations included infant stimulation, household play, dressing up, creative play, gross motor activities and shop play. The children were shown the equipment in each of these situations. If they did not respond spontaneously, they were prompted verbally and/or physically to begin to play. Adults did not remain involved once the child began to play unless the child requested their help (for example, to spin the top) or involved them in the play (for example, gave them a drink). The child's activities were recorded while interest was displayed in the toy or equipment. Recording finished when the child obviously began to repeat the same action patterns, or when the child rejected an item or pushed one away and selected a new item. Because each child's interaction with the equipment was so highly individual, an exact time limit could not be set.

Samples of play and language obtained in these situations were interpreted in relation to the abilities described on the Symbolic Play Scale (Westby, 1980). Comparisons of obtained language levels with the REEL Scale and obtained play levels with the Uzgiris and Hunt Scales provided measures of the validity of the Westby Scale as an index of the development of language and play in children with severe intellectual disabilities.

Results

Table 2-1 presents a summary of the language and play assessments for all the children in the study, providing details of the receptive, expressive and combined language ages on the REEL Scale; play and overall average score on the Uzgiris and Hunt Scales; and play and language scores on the Westby Scale.

In all assessments, language and play results show a significant developmental delay in relation to chronological age. There is no complete agreement between results on the REEL language scores and Westby language scores, with child 1, child 2 and child 6 all showing a difference as indicated in Figure 2-1. Figure 2-2 shows there are two situations reported where play results on the Uzgiris and Hunt Scales and on the Westby Scale are not the same (child 1 and child 2). These differences highlight the variable nature of formal assessments and their effects on results when used with young children with intellectual disabilities. The Westby Scale acknowledges the functional aspects of daily interactions, while the REEL Scale and Uzgiris and Hunt Scales focus more specifically on responses in given structured situations. Fewell and Kaminski (1988) referred to this problem in the use of formal assessments.

Examination of the nature of each student's profile can provide greater understanding of the language and play needs of each child. It is important to realise that such a group of students is essentially heterogeneous rather than homogeneous in nature. Therefore analysis and discussion of the results involve a series of individual trends instead of the more usual analysis of group effects.

Table 2-1: Language and play assessments on the REEL Scale, the Uzgiris and Hunt Scales and the Westby Scale.

Child	C.A.	REEL			Uzgiris and Hunt		Westby	
		R.L.A.	E.L.A.	C.L.A.	Play	Average	Play	Language
1	9y	1m	3m	2m	7m	4m	9m	9m
2	9y	11m	3m	7m	10m	9m	13–17m	13–17m
3	4y	1m	1m	1m	10m	11m	9–12m	Prior to 9m
4	7y	18m	18m	18m	19m	19m	19–22m	17–19m
5	9y	30m	30m	30m	24m	22m	24–30m	24–30m
6	9y	30m	30m	30m	19m	22m	17–19m	19–22m

Code: C.A. = Chronological age; R.L.A. = Receptive language age; E.L.A. = Expressive language age; C.L.A. = Combined language age; y = years; m = months.

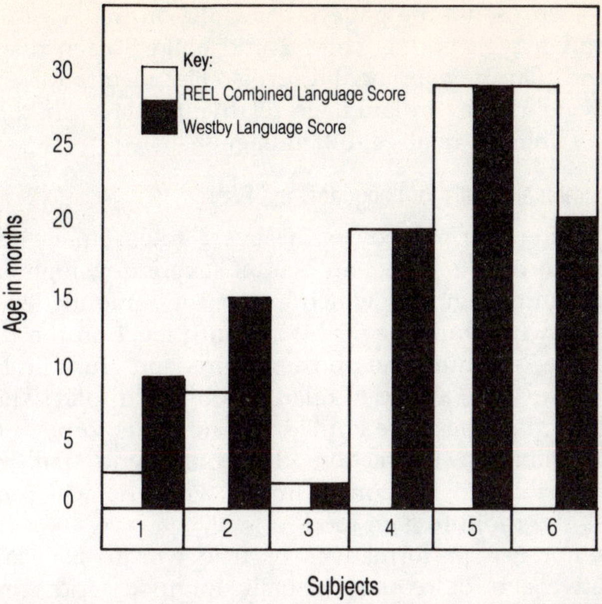

Figure 2-1: Comparison of language scores on REEL Scale and on Westby Scale.

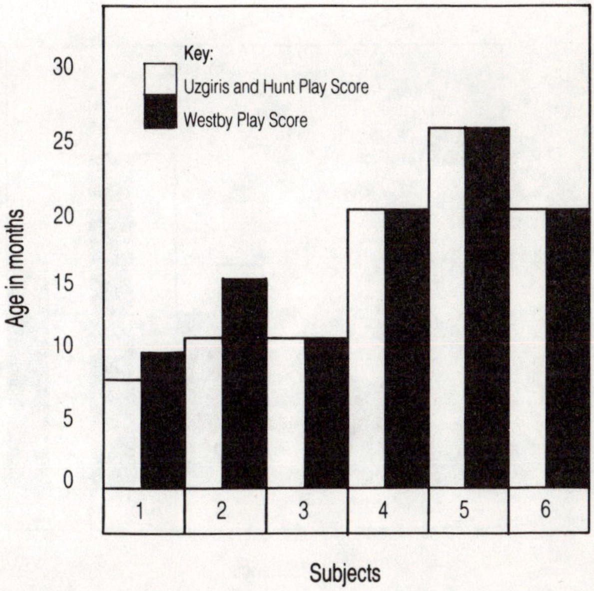

Figure 2-2: Comparison of play scores on Uzgiris and Hunt Scales and on Westby Scale.

Figure 2-3 represents the pattern of results on the Westby Scale for language and play. Child 1, child 2 and child 5 each display equal language and play developmental levels. The results for child 3 and child 4 indicate a delay in language relative to play. Child 6 shows a delay in play abilities relative to language skills.

Equal Developmental Levels for Language and Play

Child 1 is a nine-year-old boy with severe intellectual and physical disabilities. The results reflect an overall severe developmental delay in both play and language, which are at the 9-month levels on the Westby Scale, with language at the 2-month level on the REEL Scale and play at the 7-month level on the Uzgiris and Hunt Scales.

He does have some ability to relate to objects in play (shaking and pushing them), but these are limited and he tends to push toys away rather than maintain interaction. The only time that means-end behaviour is exhibited is at meal times, when he will purposefully move across the room to gain food.

He does not use performatives or true words. He can perform communicative acts of request (usually for food) and command in relation to his daily living needs. He does protest if being hurt, and undertakes some social interaction in set contexts. For example, he puts his hand out to continue the action rhyme game "roly-poly" and his head forward to repeat "peek-a-boo".

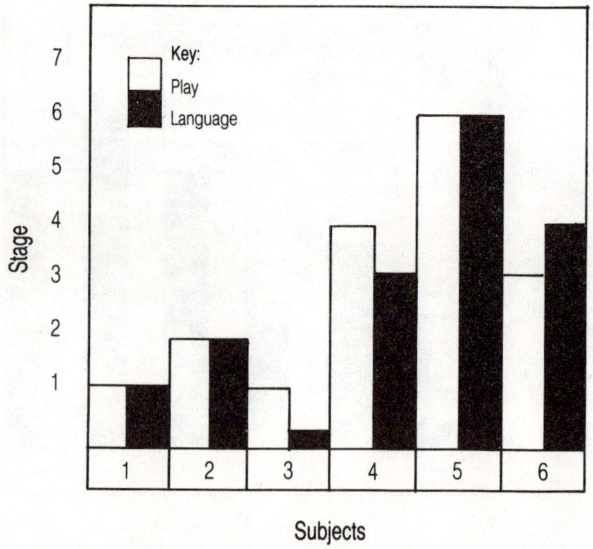

Figure 2-3: Results on the Westby Symbolic Play Scale for Play and Language. Note: Stages relate to Westby Scale age ranges (Westby, 1980).

The assessment indicates that this student needs assistance with developing social interactive skills and with communicating his needs and wants. It is also interesting to note that he responds interactively and communicatively in social games (such as peek-a-boo) and in daily care routines (such as meals). He shows little response to toys and equipment and rarely requests these. In order to teach him to communicate more effectively, intervention needs to be based at these earlier levels and to involve both the form and function of communication behaviours (Harrison et al, 1987).

Instead of play, the focus needs to be on the routines of communication in daily interaction situations, giving the student the chance to practise purposeful communicative behaviours, providing reinforcement for behaviours that he already exhibits and refining these toward more conventional gestures and vocalisations.

Assessments of both language (REEL Scale) and play skills (Uzgiris and Hunt Scales) provide results below those of the Westby Scale. This also reflects the need to assess students with severe intellectual disabilities in natural contexts, observing interactional patterns rather than the specific language and object manipulation skills that more formal measures reflect.

Child 2, also aged nine years, displays similar development in play and language. This is a student with severe intellectual disability who spends much of his time in self-stimulatory activities. His overall development on the Westby Scale is in the 13 to 17 months range, while his language score on the REEL Scale is 7 months and play score on the Uzgiris and Hunt Scales is 10 months.

In play he does explore toys to discover operations through trial and error. If he cannot make them function, he will hit and bang them and will occasionally ask for help by handing the toy to an adult or placing the adult's hand on the toy. On one occasion in the observation session he was given a rattle that can be blown to produce a squeak. He first discovered this when mouthing the toy. He looked and laughed and repeated the action. He later returned to the toy but didn't blow into the appropriate place. When he didn't get the reaction he wanted, he handed the toy to the observer who modelled the action. When it still wouldn't work for him, he banged the table and cried.

He is able to use adults as tools to gain desired results more often in relation to everyday needs. For example, he will take hold of his teacher's hand and move it to his shoe when it has come off, or to his jumper when he is told to take it off.

There is evidence of development in this boy's ability to perform communicative functions of request, command, greeting, interaction and protest, although he relies on his own set of idiosyncratic gestures.

He will look and then put his face up to one side to be kissed by his parent for a greeting. He looks in response to his name and responds appropriately to given instructions within his usual repertoire. He will come to adults in the room, touch them and look at them in the eye as if to say, "I'm still here". He takes an adult's hand to help with dressing as needed. Many of the functions performed, however, are limited to set contexts and are not always self-initiated. For example, he will not ask for a drink when needed or help with his jumper unless first told to remove it.

The other assessment results are not consistent with the results on the Westby Scale. Again, the issue relates to the appropriateness of the use of formal measures such as the REEL Scale and the Uzgiris and Hunt Scales for students with intellectual disabilities as severe as that exhibited by this student. Observations in natural settings that focus on daily interactions, as used in the Westby Scale, produce results that may be more appropriate measures of functional abilities.

While this student is developing the ability to communicate, there is not a corresponding development in vocalisation. He can continue to be trained to communicate, with the introduction of an augmentative communication system to assist where vocalisations are not present. In addition, there needs to be specific training to encourage the student's attempts to initiate communication events. Halle (1984) provides a model of naturalistic training using mand-model, delay and incidental-teaching strategies, which could be relevant to this student's needs. Given this boy's age and the nature of his disability, play may not be an appropriate means of intervention for the future, but, rather, functional interactions in natural social situations may provide a more age-appropriate means of further developing his communication skills.

Child 5, aged nine years, is the third student to exhibit similar levels on the play and language development measures, with both being at the 24 to 30 months level on the Westby Scale, which is a more advanced level than the two previous students of the same age. His language score on the REEL Scale is 30 months and play score on the Uzgiris and Hunt Scales is 24 months.

In play this boy represents daily experiences in short, isolated sequences that are true to life. He pretends to be the mum. He puts dolls into the pram and talks to them. He is also beginning to represent other people's roles. In the shopping corner, he put the fruit into a bag, the bag over his shoulder and proclaimed, "Go shopping". He took another child with him, said goodbye to each person in the room and walked to the door. He repeated this sequence but didn't ever leave the room or follow through with the shopping.

Parallel play predominates in most situations involving this child.

He will play next to but not with another child when playing with the train set. Association play is beginning to appear when he is pretending to be the mum or the teacher and when he plays in the shopping corner.

This boy is able to use language, so that a sample could be taken in play interactions. He responds to and uses "wh-" questions, and the use of "-ing", plurals and possessives is also evident.

Westby (1980) wrote that where play and language are at similar levels, then therapy should provide experiences to facilitate the development of symbolic abilities so that language skills will develop from these interaction experiences. Awareness of the level of existing skills enables language to be extended in these interactional settings. This student's play is more advanced than that of the previous students, and he demonstrates a pleasure in acting out sequences of events, with elements of pretending evident. Play therefore provides an ideal setting to model the appropriate language usages needed by this child for further development, and the opportunity for social interaction with non-disabled peers is also appropriate.

Delayed Language Development Relative to Play Abilities

Child 3 is a four-year-old student with severe intellectual disability believed to be associated with environmental deprivation. On the Westby Scale, his play level is 9 to 12 months, while language is at a level prior to 9 months. His language is reported to be at the 1-month level on the REEL Scale and his play at the 10-month level on the Uzgiris and Hunt Scales.

In play he applies a few schemes in attempts to operate toys but is basically disinterested if he does not get an immediate response. He then drops the toy and reverts to self-stimulating behaviour such as hand-flapping and shaking his head. What is significant is that he does not attempt to seek adult assistance, even if given a cue to do so.

His interaction with objects tends to be functional rather than demonstrating elements of pretend play. For example, he raised the phone to his ear, and a cup to his mouth. When presented with a toy iron, he was very purposeful in his search for appropriate articles to iron. He does not relate to dolls and drops them rather than maintaining a hold on them. While he uses most toys appropriately, he is very limited in his application of play. For example, he will lie in one place to play with a car, and his attention to play is very brief.

His language development does not register on the Westby Scale (prior to 9 months). He does not use performatives, and his only vocalisation consists of "mmm" used non-specifically and infrequently. He cries and whinges, which can be interpreted as a protest, and uses his hand to reject food items he does not know or like. He does not request or command in a communicative manner, or use specific gestures or eye contact to express these intentions. His communicative acts are at the stage where adults interpret what they think is intended, with most acts being responses to affective and primary needs.

The child attended school for only one term prior to assessment. He had attended an Early Intervention Program, where structured programming might have affected the development of higher levels of communication in some areas (Westby, 1980), while environmental deprivation continues to influence lower levels of development in the more socially relevant areas. The work of Bruner (1983) could provide a relevant approach to intervention for this student, as he emphasises the social as well as the cognitive bases for language acquisition (Westby, 1980; Harrison et al, 1987).

This child would benefit from involvement in caretaker–child types of games, where he could learn how to take turns, how to combine gaze, gestures and vocal behaviours, and how to establish, maintain or terminate an interaction. The fact that he is capable of some more advanced play abilities needs to be expanded through intervention that focuses on extending his involvement with toys.

Rather than attempting to teach him vocalisations for labels of objects, this boy needs to expand on his use of the functions of language, to learn that he can intentionally let others know what he wants. Delay procedures, as described earlier, have been recommended to assist him in developing the ability to initiate interactions. He needs also to understand and trust that there will be consistency in responses from adults, a strategy referred to earlier as contingent responding.

Child 4 also exhibits a greater delay in language than in play. Her chronological age is seven years. While this girl's physical development is normal, she has a severe intellectual disability due to unknown causes. She is functioning at 17–19 months for language and 19–22 months for play on the Westby Scale, 18 months for language on the REEL Scale and 19 months for play on the Uzgiris and Hunt Scales.

Her symbolic play extends beyond herself, as she applies schemes to dolls and adults — for example, when feeding, brushing hair and giving a drink. She also applies a single scheme to more than one object or person. For example, given a cup, she will drink some herself, give some to a doll and give some to her teacher. She combines two toys in play, such as putting the phone to the doll's ear. She still searches for objects in play, such as a spoon, not a stick or substitute, for stirring.

This child's language reflects the use of performatives to bridge the gap to labelling (Bricker & Bricker, 1974). Many of her vocalisations are performatives, representing actions and tied to the immediate context. For example, "jump" when on the trampoline, "push" with certain toys and "sup sup" for cup. She names all the children in the class and some objects. She uses words for familiar actions and is able to combine gestures and vocalisations to exhibit communicative functions.

According to Westby (1980), if play is in advance of language, then speech and language remediation is warranted. Westby suggests that therapy should begin with the language level exhibited and should provide both structured and play remediation sessions, with the primary focus on play sessions designed to elicit language skills. She recommends modelling and formal training of concepts and structures the child needs, using the strategy referred to earlier as scaffolding for communication. Incidental-teaching procedures and the mand-model technique have also been found to be effective in extending verbal abilities (Halle, 1984) and would be appropriate to include with play situations.

Delayed Play Abilities Relative to Language Development

Child 6 is a nine-year-old girl with severe intellectual disability. On the Westby Scale she is functioning at the 17–19 months level for play and 19–22 months for language. There is a higher language score reported on the REEL Scale, at 30 months, while the play score on the Uzgiris and Hunt Scales is similar to the Westby score at 19 months.

Most noticeable in this child is a repetitive return to obsessive behaviours such as poking small objects into any available space in the room (into keyholes, under cupboards, behind heaters) whenever she is left undirected. This behaviour is relevant in assessing her play development as it dominates to such an extent that she shows very little involvement in play. Despite this, she is able to pretend (when directed in play situations) and applies this ability to auto-symbolic play (17–19 months on the Westby Scale). She will pretend to drink from a doll's cup and say, "Mmm, nice milk", indicating some level of play development. Some instances of play were at a higher level; for example, she gave herself and the doll bread. She did pretend to get sugar with a spoon and put it into a cup. However, because she does not frequently become involved in play, her behaviours have not been extended and are not representative of her overall play levels.

As stated previously, her language development is at the 19–22 months level on the Westby Scale, although she also has certain abilities at higher levels. She is able to refer to objects and persons not present and combines words to express the range of semantic relations. She often asks questions, especially "where?" and "what?", but usually knows the reply. She responds appropriately to these questions in context. However, a language sample taken over several situations indicates that her vocabulary consists of several well-known phrases often used inappropriately. For example, when in the dolls' corner she asked, "Go in bus?", "Sing tape?" and "Go home mummy?" Such language resembles that of the "cocktail party syndrome" (McCormick & Schiefelbusch, 1984, p 92). That is, her chatter gives an impression of extended ability, but much of it is repetitive and out of context.

The REEL assessment provides a higher score for language than the Westby assessment, the difference again being explained by the nature of the assessment materials. While the REEL scales sample items normally found at particular age-group levels, Westby scales sample language as it is used in communicative and interactional settings. In this case, the girl's language displays more mature forms but is inappropriate to the interactional setting and the nature of communication that normally takes place in that setting.

For Child 6 language appears to have developed in advance of play. Westby (1980) found this occurred when language was used in echolalic or stereotyped ways. That appears to be true in this case. While this student can exhibit play skills at levels that match her language skills, she has to be prompted to do so and becomes aggressive if maintained in that situation. In addition, the higher-level language abilities exhibited are consistently out of context and inappropriate. If left undirected, she prefers her own idiosyncratic behaviours (poking objects into holes) to any form of play or involvement with toys. In the observation sessions, she needed prompting to become involved in playing with anything other than infant-stimulation toys of a musical kind and then played for a very short time. McHale et al (1980), in their study of autistic children, also report similar findings. They found that symbolic language usage can be more advanced than the appropriateness of the way that language is used in daily situations.

Play session evaluations indicate that Child 6 is capable of higher levels of communicative and language functioning. However, her extreme dislike of involvement in play activities makes this a questionable medium for therapy. Instead, it appears essential that the contextual appropriateness of her utterances be monitored. Only those utterances that are appropriate should be responded to and reinforced. Daily social interactions would provide the ideal times for appropriate language structures to be modelled. Social interactions with age peers who are not disabled could be used to encourage appropriate language. Her reluctance to use her free time appropriately indicates that she needs training in age-appropriate leisure activities with the use of naturalistic training strategies suggested by Halle (1984).

In conclusion, the highly individual nature of this student's responses highlights the need to assess actual performance variables of language and play in natural interactive situations. It is important to assess the performance of early communicative functions, as for some students this may be the level of their abilities even if they are older in chronological age. The Westby Scale provides a relevant assessment tool for levels of language development and the appropriateness of language used. The play scale indicates the levels of symbolic abilities that are relevant to language.

Play as the basis of therapy proves an ideal means to develop the necessary language and cognitive skills in young children. However, for students with greater degrees of difference between chronological age and performance age, functional language usage during daily routines and age-appropriate leisure activities provides a more relevant basis for implementing naturalistic interventions. "Thus the study of the development of play clearly has both theoretical significance as well as practical implications for intervention with handicapped youngsters" (Fewell & Kaminski, 1988, p 145).

Implications for Classroom Practices

An awareness of the child's level of cognitive development, as evidenced by symbolic play abilities, enables the educator to direct intervention through play in order to achieve specific goals of language development. Importance is placed on naturalistic processes of learning, where play provides a natural medium for children to practise and extend such processes. Observations in natural settings can enable both play and language development levels to be assessed. These provide an understanding of a student's functioning level.

The use of standardised measures for students with severe intellectual disabilities can create problems when these tests do not sample early social communicative acts. The idiosyncratic nature of communicative responses in these children and the heterogeneous nature of the total population need to be recognised and acknowledged by any assessment method. In the present study these difficulties were addressed through the use of an alternative assessment approach.

Based on observations in natural contexts, this study indicates some generalised treatment principles that can be applied to language intervention for students with severe intellectual disabilities. Each situation observed, clearly indicated that intervention based on play alone is not sufficient to enable language to develop. Specific intervention aimed at extending language skills through play is necessary.

Such intervention can be unobtrusive and child-centred when based on the strategies described earlier.

When a student's language and play abilities are at similar levels and are not significantly delayed in relation to age, then intervention based on play will lead to the interactive experiences needed to facilitate the development of both cognitive and language skills. For students with severe cognitive and language delays, intervention needs to focus on daily interaction situations that elicit the use of functional communication.

Where there is evidence of the use of early communicative functions and play is in advance of language, then intervention needs to begin by assessing the language skills needed for play routines and structuring the environment to elicit these skills. For students who have not developed early communicative functions but are exhibiting progress in play skills, the focus of intervention should be on the quality of social interactions and caretaker games.

Where a student's language development appears to be in advance of play, it is important to examine the appropriateness of the language used in relation to the situation and the nature of the play skills normally exhibited. Both may in fact be rather stereotyped and repetitive. Intervention to extend play sequences can assist the student to develop beyond such simple routines. However, if the student's behaviour persists with increasing age, then the focus needs to shift toward ensuring the appropriateness of social interactions in daily care situations.

In evaluating the use of an assessment procedure such as the Westby Scale, which focuses on observations of play and language usage in natural situations, both positive and negative features can be seen. Positive features include the observation of natural situations as a basis for assessment information; the recognition of communication abilities that are used in interactions and that may exist prior to the use of words; and the provision of an intervention model for young students with intellectual disabilities focusing on the process of learning in natural contexts.

However, the limits of these assessment procedures also need to be acknowledged. The inappropriateness of play as an intervention strategy for older students has already been discussed. There is also very little information given by Westby assessments to guide intervention decisions for students with a functional level earlier than nine months, which is the necessary level for intervention to begin for many students with a severe intellectual disability.

Play is the natural learning context for young children. In play they develop their own understanding of the environment at a rate that they can master. Their developing ability to act on the environment makes children increasingly independent. For students who lack this ability, learned helplessness may become an issue (Romski, Sevcik & Joyner, 1984). It becomes easier for caregivers to anticipate a student's needs and to satisfy them without expecting the student to initiate a communicative act indicating those desires. However, if the caretaker is able to structure the environment by using incidental intervention strategies during play to encourage the initiation of communication and responding behaviours in the child, then progress may be made in the development of communicative abilities. For example, strategies may include the offering of choices at mealtimes, the use of delay procedures in normal routines, placing a desired object out of reach or placing an object in an unexpected context.

The ability to communicate with others and share play experiences with non-disabled peers is important to the acceptance of students with developmental disabilities in integrated settings. An approach that focuses on play to assist in language development also provides an ideal means for students to increase their acceptance by and ability to interact with others. "Play can be a very powerful means of enhancing normalisation and helping the child to develop within the family, the classroom, and the community" (Musselwhite, 1986, p 12).

Increasing the student's ability to engage in symbolic play requires careful planning, involving observation of the student's play levels, provision of materials appropriate to those levels and involvement with the student in play. For example, if the student is still at the stage of looking for like objects to represent the real object, then it is important to provide these and also similar representations. There is little to be gained by introducing miniature objects for play if the student is still at the stage of using life-size objects. Relating observations to the Westby Scale can indicate when a student is approaching the time when objects at the next level can be introduced.

Students with intellectual disabilities will benefit from the structured enactment of events that normal children usually participate in. If the student is beginning to sequence events, then the provision of additional materials and the enactment of a common sequence of events can be structured. For example, a birthday party with peers using a real cake or with dolls and a pretend cake. Carefully structured interventions in play should assist the child to be involved in the process of learning rather than directing that learning beyond the child's own mental capacities. Fein (1975, p 295) indicated that ". . . children imitate that which they can already understand and that transformations arise from sources other than children's imitation of playful adults."

Earlier discussion referred to scaffolding for play and language as a means of gradually extending the child beyond existing ability levels.

Such strategies are unobtrusive and avoid situations where the adult is too directive. Learning through play needs to be a child-centred process.

Conclusions

The fact that an orderly sequence in the development of symbolic play skills has been identified and parallel development in language abilities has been mapped provides a natural basis for the assessment of cognitive and language abilities, just as the assessment of other abilities in early childhood is based on similar sequences of development. For example, the assessment of gross motor abilities is based on functional stages in the development of movement patterns in normal infants.

It is well known that play provides a necessary means for normal infants to explore and understand their world and to acquire increasing control over that environment (Fewell & Kaminski, 1988). Research indicates that intellectually disabled students display similar patterns of play development as those found in normally developing infants, although developmental ages vary with the individual's disability. Similar results were reflected in the present study.

Curriculum development for young students with intellectual disabilities addresses such domains as fine motor and gross motor skills, cognitive, personal and social development, and language abilities. The need to develop functional independence and readiness to learn formal skills can limit the extent to which play is included in the curriculum. However, play integrates all aspects of learning in the early years and provides a natural means to assess developmental levels and to intervene with instructional strategies.

It is believed that the ability to symbolise provides a common underlying ability for the development of both play and language skills. In monitoring the development of the ability to symbolise, importance is placed on basing the assessment on observations of the child in natural settings. Moreover, naturalistic intervention strategies are used to address deficits in play or language abilities and to continually extend existing skills.

While limited in size, the reported study does reflect different patterns of development, with some students obtaining the same score on both language and play development but at various levels. The Westby Scale indicates the need to focus on developing communicative functions through gestures prior to speech. For students with a more severe intellectual disability, this provides an important area for further research. Do developmental patterns of early communicative intent in normal children provide an appropriate measure for communication development in students with severe intellectual disabilities? Do these abilities also need to be developed in the intellectually disabled population prior to the use of an alternative language system, where signing or pictures may be used to assist communication or to substitute for spoken words?

The study questions the appropriateness of play for older students with more severe intellectual disabilities. Play represents a form of natural intervention for young students and provides an ideal opportunity for both assessment and intervention programs for communication and language development. For older students, daily care activities and leisure skill programs provide a means for maintaining intervention that is functional and appropriate.

There is a developmental interdependence between play and language, with symbolic ability providing a common link. Symbolic ability normally develops as an outcome of the first two years of social interaction and sensorimotor cognitive development. Thus both the cognitive and social qualities of the child's early life play an important role in the development of prelinguistic skills, the acquisition of a language system and the communicative use of that system.

References

Atlas, J.A. & Lapidus, B.L. (1988). Symbolization levels in communicative behaviors of children showing pervasive developmental disorders. *Journal of Communication Disorders 21*, 75–84.

Bates, E. (1979). *The emergence of symbols: Cognition and communication in infancy*. New York: Academic Press.

Bates, E., Camaioni, L. & Volterra, V. (1975). The acquisition of performatives prior to speech. *Merrill-Palmer Quarterly 21 (3)*, 205–26.

Beeghly, M., Weiss-Perry, B. & Cicchetti, D. (1989). Beyond sensorimotor functioning: Early communicative and play development of children with Down syndrome. In D. Cicchetti & M. Beeghly (eds), *Children with Down syndrome: A developmental perspective*. New York: Cambridge University Press.

Bloom, L. (1970). *Language development: Form and function in emerging grammars*. Cambridge: M.I.T. Press.

Bloom, L. & Lahey, M. (1978). *Language development and language disorders*. New York: John Wiley & Sons.

Bowerman, M.F. (1978). Semantic and syntactic development. In R.L. Schiefelbusch (ed.), *Bases of language intervention*. Baltimore: University Park Press.

Bricker, W.A. & Bricker, D.D. (1974). An early language training strategy. In R.L. Schiefelbusch & L.R. Lloyd (eds), *Language perspectives: Acquisition, retardation and intervention*. Baltimore: University Park Press.

Bruner, J.S. (1983). *Child's talk: Learning to use language*. London: Oxford University Press.

Butterfield, N., Arthur, M. & Linfoot, K. (1992). Meeting teacher needs in communication programming for students with severe intellectual disability: The Creating Communicative Contexts Manual, *Special Education Perspectives 1 (1)*, 35–43.

Bzoch, K.R. & League, R. (1978). *Assessing language skills in infancy*. Baltimore: University Park Press.

Corrigan, R. (1982). The control of animate and inanimate components in pretend play and language. *Child Development 53 (5)*, 1343–53.

Dunst, C.J. (1980). *A clinical and educational manual for use with the Uzgiris and Hunt Scales of Infant Psychological Development*. Baltimore: University Park Press.

Dunst, C.J. & Lowe, L.W. (1986). From reflex to symbol: Describing, explaining and fostering communicative competence. *Augmentative and Alternative Communication 2 (1)*, 11–18.

Fein, G.G. (1975). A transactional analysis of pretending. *Developmental Psychology 11*, 155–416.

Fewell, R.R. & Kaminski, R. (1988). Play skill development and instruction for young children with handicaps. In S.L. Odom & M.B. Karnes (eds), *Early intervention for infants and children with handicaps*. Baltimore: Paul H. Brookes.

Halle, J.W. (1984). Arranging the natural environment to occasion language: Giving severely language-delayed children reasons to communicate. *Seminars in Speech and Language 5 (3)*, 185–97.

Halle, J.W., Marshall, A.M. & Spradlin, J.E. (1979). Time delay: A technique to increase language use and facilitate generalization in retarded children. *Journal of Applied Behavior Analysis 12*, 431–39.

Halliday, M.A.K. (1975). *Learning how to mean: Explorations in the development of language*. Columbus: Charles E. Merrill.

Harrison, D., Lombardino, L.J. & Stapell, J.B. (1987). The development of early communication: Using developmental literature for selecting communication goals. *The Journal of Special Education 20 (4)*, 463–73.

Hart, B.M. & Risley, T.R. (1968). Establishing use of descriptive adjectives in the spontaneous speech of disadvantaged preschool children. *Journal of Applied Behavior Analysis 1*, 109–20.

Kangas, K.A. & Lloyd, L.L. (1988). Early cognitive skills as prerequisites to augmentative and alternative communication use: What are we waiting for? *Augmentative and Alternative Communication 4 (4)*, 211–21.

Kennedy, M.D., Sheridan, M.K., Radlinski, S.H. & Beeghly, M. (1991). Play-language relationships in young children with developmental delays: Implications for assessment. *Journal of Speech and Hearing Research 34*, 112–22.

Leibergott, J. & Swope, S. (1976). Play as a base for language acquisition. In F.B. Withrow & C.J. Nygren (eds), *Language, materials and curriculum management for the handicapped learner*. Columbus: Charles E. Merrill.

Linder, T.W. (1993). *Transdisciplinary play-based assessment* (rev. edn). Baltimore: Paul H. Brookes.

Lowe, M. (1975). Trends in the development of representational play in infants from one to three years: An observational study. *Journal of Child Psychology and Psychiatry 16*, 33–47.

McCormick, L. & Schiefelbusch, R. (1984). *Early language intervention: An introduction*. Columbus: Charles E. Merrill.

McCormick, L. & Shane, H. (1984). Augmentative communication. In L.L.

McCormick & R.L. Schiefelbusch (eds), *Early language intervention*. Columbus: Charles E. Merrill.

McCune-Nicholich, L. (1981). Towards symbolic functioning: Structure of early pretend games and potential parallels with language. *Child Development 52*, 785–97.

McCune-Nicholich, L. & Carol, S. (1981). Development of symbolic play: Implications for the language specialist. *Topics in Language Disorders 2*, 1–15.

McHale, S.M., Simeonsson, R.J., Marcus, L.M. & Olley, J.G. (1980). The social and symbolic quality of autistic children's communication. *Journal of Autism and Developmental Disorders 10 (3)*, 299–311.

McLean, J.E. & Snyder-McLean, L.K. (1978). *A transactional approach to early language training*. Columbus: Charles E. Merrill.

McLean, J. & Snyder-McLean, L. (1987). Form and function of communicative behaviour among persons with severe developmental disabilities. *Australia and New Zealand Journal of Developmental Disabilities 13 (2)*, 83–98.

Morehead, D.M. & Morehead, A. (1974). From signal to sign: A Piagetian view of thought and language during the first two years. In R.L. Schiefelbusch & L.R. Lloyd (eds), *Language perspectives: Acquisition, retardation and intervention*. Baltimore: University Park Press.

Mundy, P., Sigman, M., Ungerer, J. & Sherman, T. (1987). Nonverbal communication and play correlates of language development in autistic children. *Journal of Autism and Developmental Disorders 17 (3)*, 349–64.

Musselwhite, C.R. (1986). *Adaptive play for special needs children*. San Diego: College Hill Press.

Owens, R.E. (1984). *Language development: An introduction*. Columbus: Charles E. Merrill.

Piaget, J. (1962). *Play, dreams and imitation in childhood*. New York: W. Norton.

Reichle, J. & Karlan, G. (1985). The selection of an augmentative system in communication intervention: A critique of decision rules. *Journal of the Association for Persons with Severe Handicaps 10 (3)*, 146–56.

Rice, M.L. (1983). Contemporary accounts of the cognition/language relationship: Implications for speech-language clinicians. *Journal of Speech and Hearing Disorders 48*, 347–59.

Rice, M.L. (1986). Mismatched premise of the communicative competence model and language intervention. In R.L. Schiefelbusch (ed.), *Language competence: Assessment and intervention*. London: Taylor & Francis.

Rice, M.L. & Kemper, S. (1984). *Child language and cognition*. Baltimore: University Park Press.

Rogers, S.J. (1977). Characteristics of the cognitive development of profoundly retarded children. *Child Development 48*, 837–43.

Rogers-Warren, A. & Warren, S. (1980). Mands for verbalization: Facilitating the display of newly trained language in children. *Behavior Modification 4*, 361–82.

Romski, M.A., Sevcik, R.A. & Joyner, S.E. (1984). Nonspeech communication systems: Implications for language intervention with mentally retarded children. *Topics in Language Disorders 5 (1)*, 66–81.

Siegel-Causey, E. & Guess, D. (1989). *Enhancing nonsymbolic communication interactions among learners with severe disabilities*. Baltimore: Paul H. Brookes.

Sinclair, H. (1973). Language acquisition and cognitive development. In T.

Moore (ed.), *Cognitive development and the acquisition of language*. New York: Academic Press.

Snyder-McLean, L., McLean, J. & Etter, R. (1988). Clinical assessment of sensorimotor knowledge in nonverbal, severely retarded clients. *Topics in Language Disorders 8 (4)*, 1–22.

Sugarman, S. (1984). The development of preverbal communication. In R.L. Schiefelbusch & S. Pickar (eds), *Communicative competence: Acquisition and intervention*. Baltimore: University Park Press.

Ungerer, J.A. & Sigman, M. (1984). The relation of play and sensorimotor behaviour to language in the second year. *Child Development 55*, 1448–55.

Warren, S. & Kaiser, A.P. (1988). Research in early language intervention. In S.L. Odom & M.B. Karnes (eds), *Early intervention for infants and children with handicaps*. Baltimore: Paul H. Brookes.

Warren, S. & Rogers-Warren, A.K. (eds) (1985). *Teaching functional language*. Texas: Pro-Ed.

Westby, C.E. (1980). Assessment of cognitive and language abilities through play. *Language Speech and Hearing Services in Schools 11*, 154–68.

Wetherby A. & Prizant B. (1990). *Communication and behavior scales. Research edition.* Chicago: Riverside Publishing.

Chapter 3

Requesting Behaviours of Preschool Children with Mild Developmental Disabilities

Diana Messervy

Bayview Heights Community Kindergarten
Cairns, Queensland

Children with mild intellectual and other developmental disabilities are being enrolled in mainstream preschools and elementary or primary schools in increasing numbers. Successful integration involves more than purely academic progress. For the integration experience to be successful, these children need to be able to interact socially with their peers. Some researchers have found that children with mild developmental delay appear to have difficulties with social interactions. Cooper (1986) observed that "these children often do not seem to fit in with their peers" (p 1). Functional social interaction requires the ability to communicate effectively. Given that many young children with mild developmental delay have accompanying language delay, the question of whether social interaction with their peers is being affected by difficulties in the area of communication needs to be considered.

Although some children may demonstrate delay in the development of the form and content of their language (Bloom & Lahey, 1978), this does not necessarily mean that they are unable to communicate effectively in order to achieve their goals. Effective communication involves proficiency in the functions of language and the use of language in a social context and is referred to as pragmatics (Bates, 1976a).

The investigation described in this chapter is concerned with pragmatic aspects of language development and draws on recent developmental theory stressing the socially interactive nature of language and language development.

A number of authors have investigated the development of pragmatic skills in young children, but few have been concerned with children who are developmentally delayed (Bates, 1976a; Cooper, 1986). There is an obvious need to add to existing knowledge about how developmentally delayed young children use the basic pragmatic language functions. However, if this knowledge is to be applied to the development of educational programs for developmentally delayed children, it is equally important to investigate this area in normally developing children. Bernard-Opitz (1982, p 109) makes the point that "With increased knowledge of the pragmatic performance of normal communicators, we will be able to specify further therapy targets for disturbed communicators." In comparing the behaviour of delayed children with their normal peers, areas of difficulty (if they exist) can be isolated and training programs developed.

Previous research has concentrated on the development of children's pragmatic language functions in their interactions with adults (Bloom & Lahey, 1978; Bruner, 1975, 1981; Cross, 1977; Newport, Gleitman & Gleitman, 1977; Norris & Hoffman, 1980; Snow, 1977; Tiegerman & Siperstein, 1984). However, to help developmentally delayed students derive maximum benefit from integrated educational experience, a major focus of future studies needs to be the investigation of the children's communications with their peers. Field (1980) found that children's early communications progress from behaviours directed to self, then to an adult, to a toy and finally to peers.

Communicative acts have a purpose or function. Halliday (1975) identified seven major functions of communication that emerge during the preschool years. His first two functions are the instrumental ("I want") and the regulatory ("Do as I tell you") functions. The mastery of the regulatory function is considered to be one of the essential steps in the developmental process (Halliday, 1975) and an essential function for healthy social existence (Schiefelbusch, 1980). Requesting falls into both the regulatory and instrumental pragmatic categories. Children initially employ nonverbal means for requesting, and gradually develop verbal strategies (Moerk, 1977; Ochs & Schieffelin, 1983; Owens, 1988; Wood, 1981). Children's verbal requests develop from direct, to indirect, to inferred forms (Bates, 1976b; Ervin-Tripp, 1980; Garvey, 1975; Wood, 1981).

Requesting develops early and is considered a "primary" pragmatic function. Cooper (1986) observed that the developmentally delayed children in her study interacted with other children in the free play situation only when they wanted a toy that another child had. Thus the development of the request function makes a logical starting point in an intervention program, both for developmental and motivational reasons.

The request function lends itself to observational investigations. Because the request function requires some overt response from the listener, it provides a directly observable means of assessing the effectiveness of the communication.

Guralnick and Groom (1985) and Beveridge et al (1988) emphasised that children's social interactions can be influenced by different situational factors. Beveridge et al pointed to a need to study the pragmatics of language for individual children in different situations to discover why children are more successful in some situations than others.

Developmentally delayed children in mainstream preschools need to be able to use the request function in their natural play situations. As social context is an integral part of pragmatic language, it would seem appropriate to observe children in their naturally occurring play situations in preschools rather than in artificial settings.

In mainstream preschool settings, communications with peers take place in many different group situations. Preschool children need to be able to communicate effectively with peers on an individual basis as well as in small and large group situations. Natural play groupings in preschools tend to consist of either two individuals playing together or a small group of three, four or five children involved in play. Therefore it is important to ascertain whether children of this age are equally effective at requesting in one-to-one situations and in small group settings. One might assume that because requests directed to adults tend to be of the one-to-one variety, children would be more adept in this setting. The small group situation appears to contain more distractions and hurdles to communication for both the communicator and the communicative partner. If it were found to be the case that preschool children are more effective in the one-to-one situation, then intervention programs could first concentrate on mastery of the request function in the individual situation and then proceed to mastery in a small group setting. If delayed children were found to be experiencing specific difficulties in either of the settings, the focus of the intervention programs could be established accordingly.

The question of whether the development of pragmatic language skills in developmentally delayed children is qualitatively or merely quantitatively different remains an issue. Some studies have found that children with developmental delay tend to interact less with peers, to be less dominant than their normally developing peers, and to be deficient in the production of verbal responses (Cooper, 1986; Kamhi & Masterson, 1988; Owens, 1988; Snyder, 1975). This appears to point to the possibility of a qualitative difference in the development of pragmatic skills in this population. However, Owens and MacDonald (1982) found that delayed children used normal pragmatic skills. According to Prutting and Kirchner (1983), the majority of studies investigating pragmatic language abilities in language-disordered children suggest they follow the same strategies as normal children at the same linguistic age.

Literature on the development of the requesting function in young developmentally delayed children in interactions with peers leaves many of these questions without definitive answers. Further research on the development of pragmatic functions in this population should indicate whether these children are in fact demonstrating a noticeably different pattern of development in pragmatic skills, or whether their language differences merely reflect a normal, albeit delayed, developmental pattern.

Successful communication by young children with peers requires both the use of a variety of communicative behaviours and congruence between verbal and nonverbal behaviours and the function of the communication (Atkinson, 1979; Lucas, 1980; Mueller, 1972; Ochs & Schieffelin, 1983; Wood, 1981). It was hypothesised in the present study that a comparison of the behaviours of normal and delayed preschoolers in relation to these factors could determine whether the children with developmental delays were experiencing difficulty in the pragmatics of communication and that it might provide information leading to the development of teaching programs for them.

The current study was planned to investigate the behaviours that normal and delayed preschool children use in their requests for a toy from peers. It was intended that findings from this study might contribute to the question concerning quantitative versus qualitative differences between the pragmatic language skills of normally developing and delayed preschool children. Another purpose of the study was to investigate the competence and dominance of developmentally delayed preschool children compared with their normally developing peers in their interactions with other children. A further aim was to determine whether the delayed children employ fewer verbal communicative strategies, and to investigate the congruence of verbal and nonverbal behaviours with the request function. Finally, the study set out to observe the effect of different sizes of play groups on the requesting behaviour of preschool children.

Methodology

Sample

The subjects were ten preschool children aged between four and a half and five and a half years of age, all attending regular preschool classes in a country town in the state of New South Wales. The children attended three preschools in the town. Five developmentally delayed children were matched with five same age, same sex peers. Two pairs of subjects were girls and three pairs were boys. Each of the pairs attended the same preschool group, so that they were well acquainted with each other and the other children in their observation groups.

The five developmentally delayed children met the following selection criteria: they all interacted with peers to some extent; they had all been observed to use the requesting function directed toward adults but had not been observed to use the request function effectively with peers without adult help; all were likely to require some in-school special education support when ultimately enrolled in kindergarten of the local primary school. Major characteristics of the subjects are shown in Table 3-1.

Procedures

The children were observed in their regular preschool classrooms in two contexts:

Table 3-1: Description of subjects and disability characteristics.

Subjects	Age	Disability	IQ levels
1D	5y 2m	Brain damage sustained at birth from difficult delivery	WPPSI Verbal 87 Perf. 64 Full Scale 74
1N	5y 3m		
2D	5y 4m	Developmental delay, unknown origin	MSCA General Cognitive Scale 72
2N	5y 4m		
3D	5y 4m	Developmental delay, unknown origin. Mother has mild intellectual disability	Binet 82
3N	5y 4m		
4D	5y 2m	Dubowitz' syndrome, a congenital disorder involving mild intellectual disability*	Binet 64
4N	5y 2m		
5D	4y 7m	Developmental delay involving language and cognitive development	Unable or unwilling to perform assessment tasks
5N	4y 8m		

Code: WPPSI refers to Wechsler Preschool and Primary Scales of Intelligence.
MSCA refers to McCarthy Scales of Children's Abilities.
Binet refers to Stanford Binet Intelligence Scale, 3rd revision, 1974 norms.
N refers to normally developing children.
D refers to children with delayed development.
*From Smith (1982).

1. Play with one child
2. Play in a group of three to four children.

The two contexts observed were chosen to discover whether the size of the group had an effect on requesting behaviour. Each subject was observed three times for approximately five minutes, in each of the two situations.

Observations were recorded using a video camera during free play sessions in the classrooms of the three preschools. The children were filmed for approximately six minutes, and data were obtained from the last five minutes of each filming session.

The event used to elicit the requesting function was the introduction of a novel toy. Only one toy was placed on the table in front of the children at any one time. The teacher placed the toy on the table, demonstrated its use once and then placed the toy in the middle of the table ensuring that it was not given to any one child. Usually that toy sustained the interest of the children for the duration of the five-minute observation period. If the children lost interest in the toy during the observation period, the teacher either demonstrated another way of using the toy or substituted another toy, using the same procedure. The toys used were: a wind-up swimming frog; a "slinky" (a large, loose spring made from plastic-covered coiled wire); a snow dome (a diorama in an enclosed liquid-filled glass container that can be inverted to release small white flakes which then settle over the scene like snow); a windmill; a set of pop-up rings on a stick; a mouthorgan; and a magnet with a variety of metal and non-metal objects.

Controlling the event in which the request function was to be observed provided uniform conditions for all subjects and minimised the problem of collecting a large amount of irrelevant data in order to observe the desired language function.

The introduction of a novel toy is an event that happens quite frequently in the normal course of the day at preschool, so that the event used to elicit the request was in keeping with the naturalistic nature of the observation.

Time sampling observations of each subject's possession of the toy were made after every thirty seconds of each five-minute observation period. Requesting behaviours were recorded and transcribed on a pre-coded raw data sheet for analysis.

A checklist of behaviours found by former research studies to be both frequently used and significant in terms of outcome was devised. This checklist (which was revised after trial observations described below) formed the basis of the raw data sheets used to transcribe observational data. Linguistic, paralinguistic and non-linguistic behaviours were recorded, as well as the devices used to gain the listener's attention.

Recording of linguistic behaviour included a transcript of all words used to request a toy. The form of the request was also noted. The work of Bates (1976b), Bates et al (1979), Garvey (1975), Ervin-Tripp (1980) and Wood (1981) suggests that young children progress from direct to indirect, explicit to less explicit and simple to complex in the forms of request used. Moerk (1977), Wood (1981), Ochs and Schieffelin (1983) and Owens (1988) refer to a developmental hierarchy in which children initially rely on nonverbal behaviours and gradually progress to the use of words with supplementary gestures. An aim of this investigation was to determine whether a difference existed between the two groups of subjects in the nonverbal and verbal forms of request used, and whether the size of the group affected the relative sophistication of the form used.

Nonverbal forms included physical (non-vocal body language such as gesture, gaze and so on) and non-word vocalisation. Verbal forms included the imperative, declarative and question forms from the "Check-list of Pragmatic Skills" devised by Cooper (1986). Other verbal forms observed in our subjects' behaviour during trial observations were included. These were: single words; indirect requests (for example, "I know some good tricks with that"); and other verbalisations (words accompanying a request but not related to the request).

Paralinguistic features such as intonation, pitch and volume, mentioned as factors involved in successful communication (Lucas, 1980; Wood, 1981), were included in the checklist. The data on intonation were not used in the ultimate analysis of results due to the unacceptably low rate of inter-observer agreement.

Nonverbal behaviours used to gain the listener's attention, such as gesture, movement of subjects in relation to the listener or toy, body position, direction of gaze and facial expression, were found to be significant in successful communication by young children with peers (Kendon & Cook, 1979; Lucas, 1980; Mueller, 1972; Ochs & Schieffelin, 1983). The nonverbal behaviours of the subjects in this investigation were thus observed and recorded under these headings.

Mueller found that the use of vocalisation or verbalisation in combination with nonverbal techniques to gain the listener's attention was crucial to communicative success. Forms of attention-seeking devices used by the subjects in this investigation were classified as: physical; non-word vocalisation; verbal; combination of vocalisation and physical; and combination of verbalisation and physical.

Data were analysed to observe the effects on requesting behaviour of:

1. group size (one child as play partner versus small group of children as play partners)
2. group characteristics (non-delayed versus delayed).

A trial of the planned data collection procedures was conducted, consisting of six observations with four target children. This was done in order to: familiarise the children with the video camera; test the coding format for transcribing the observations and alter it if necessary; test whether the planned event did in fact elicit the request function; and test whether the types of toys introduced were in fact effective in motivating children to request.

Following the trial, some revisions of the data sheet were found to be necessary. An item from the original taxonomy of behaviours was deleted as the result of the trial. This concerned the visual attention of the communicative partner to the communicator. Some additional behaviours within the existing categories were also observed during the trial and were subsequently added to the raw data sheet.

During the trial observations it was found that the event of introducing a toy, and the types of toys used, did in fact elicit the request function in the children observed.

An unexpected finding from the trial observations was the influence of gender on behaviour and outcomes. In all except one preschool, girls were effective when communicating with other girls but were very much less successful when boys were part of the group. The boys tended to dominate. For this reason, it was decided that, in the preschools where this behaviour was observed, groups would be of a single sex composition.

A second observer independently scored 20% of the observations. Inter-observer agreement for the transcription of behaviours from the video to the data sheets was calculated by using a point-by-point percentage of agreement formula (Bernard-Opitz, 1982, p 102). A training session was conducted, and information about the data sheets and criteria for scoring observations were given in writing to the second observer.

Each behaviour category was analysed separately to ascertain those behaviours that were most frequently used and the influence of group size and developmental level on behaviours. Outcomes of requests were analysed in terms of group size and developmental level. Four behaviour categories (strategies to gain the listener's attention, gesture, verbal form and direction of gaze) were compared with outcomes to identify any connections between certain behaviour patterns and outcomes. These data were analysed in terms of the subjects' developmental level.

The small number of subjects used in this study certainly limits the extent to which generalisations can be made from the results. However, results for these subjects, in these particular contexts, can be treated with confidence for the following reasons. There is a relatively large amount of data on the behaviour of these children, taken from 60 five-minute observations in total, resulting in 340 identified requests for a toy. Favourable rates of inter-observer and intra-observer agreement add to the reliability of the data (see Tables 3-2 and 3-3).

Results

Number of Requests

The number of requests made by the subjects was not greatly affected by group size, although there were slightly more requests made in the larger group context (176) than in the one-to-one situation (164). Similarly, developmental level had a negligible effect on the number of requests made, the delayed group making only slightly more requests than the normal group (171:169).

Figure 3-1 presents the number of requests made by each individual in the matched pairs of subjects. It can be seen that the number of requests made by individuals varied markedly and ranged from no requests at all from subject 3 of the delayed group (3D) to 59 requests made by subject 4 from the normal group (4N). The members of the pairs of subjects 1, 4 and 5 made similar numbers of requests, although subjects 3D and 3N both made the smallest number of requests of their developmental groups.

Table 3-2: Rate of *inter-observer* agreement for the occurrence of requests for a toy and for other aspects of requesting behaviour.

Item	Agreement
Occurrence of requests	88%
Transcript of words	78%
Form of requests	86%
Intonation	45%
Voice pitch	90%
Voice volume	92%
Gesture	80%
Outcome	87%
Movement	82%
Body orientation	84%
Direction of gaze	88%
Facial expression	87%
Strategies	99%
Possession of toy	100%

Table 3-3: Rate of *intra-observer* agreement for the occurrence of requests for a toy and for other aspects of requesting behaviour.

Item	Agreement
Occurrence of requests	97%
Transcript of words	86%
Form of requests	92%
Intonation	79%
Voice pitch	100%
Voice volume	89%
Gesture	92%
Outcome	92%
Movement	85%
Body orientation	96%
Direction of gaze	90%
Facial expression	100%
Strategies	100%
Possession of toy	100%

Requesting Behaviours

Table 3-4 shows the most common behaviours used to request a toy by all the subjects. The most frequent strategy used to gain the listener's attention was the verbal/physical combination, followed by physical strategies. Questions, imperatives and declaratives were the most commonly used forms of request, in that order. Moderate pitch and volume were far more frequently observed than high and low pitch and volume. The gestures most frequently used were attempting to take the toy from another child, and touching or pulling the toy. All subjects moved toward the child with the toy most frequently. In many instances, no movement was noted. A forward body posture and less often an erect posture were the most frequently noted body orientations. Most subjects looked toward the toy and a neutral facial expression was seen far more frequently than any other.

Effects of Group Size

Group size was found to have a major effect on the amount of time the subjects had possession of the toys and on the outcome of requests. The larger group size presented more difficulties for all subjects in terms of time in possession of the toy and of outcome of requests.

Figure 3-2 shows the effect of group size on rates of possession of toy. (Group size A denotes the one-to-one situation, while group size B denotes the small group situation.) In the one-to-one situation the subjects had possession of the toy 43% of the time, compared with 23% of the time in the larger group situation.

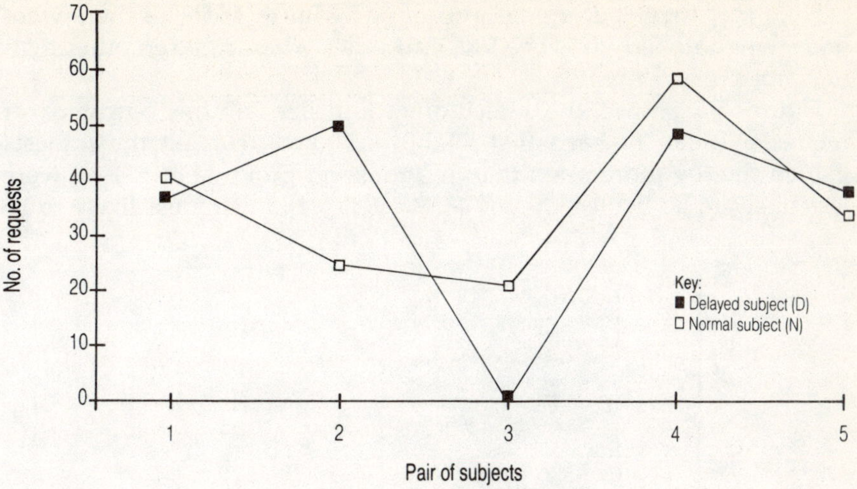

Figure 3-1: Number of requests from individual subjects.

Table 3-4: Most common requesting behaviours.

Feature	Behaviour				
Strategy:	Verbal and physical	Physical		Other	Total
%	47	37		16	100
Form:	Question	Imperative	Declarative	Other	Total
%	32.5	22.5	16.5	28.5	100
Voice pitch:	Moderate			Other	Total
%	84			16	100
Voice volume:	Moderate			Other	Total
%	77.5			22.5	100
Gesture:	Touch/pull toy	Take toy		Other	Total
%	26	32.5		41.5	100
Direction of movement:	Toward self	Static		Other	Total
%	54	40		6	100
Body orientation:	Inclined forward	Erect		Other	Total
%	58.5	31		10.5	100
Direction of gaze:	Toward toy			Other	Total
%	67			33	100
Facial expression:	Neutral	Smile		Other	Total
%	51	20		29	100

Note that these percentages do not add up to 100% as there were times when nobody had the toy, and times when children other than the subjects had the toy.

Figure 3-3 shows the effect of group size on the outcomes of requests. It can be seen that in the one-to-one context the subjects gained the toy more often than in the larger group (43% : 24%); were less likely to be denied the toy (35% : 49%); and were less likely to be

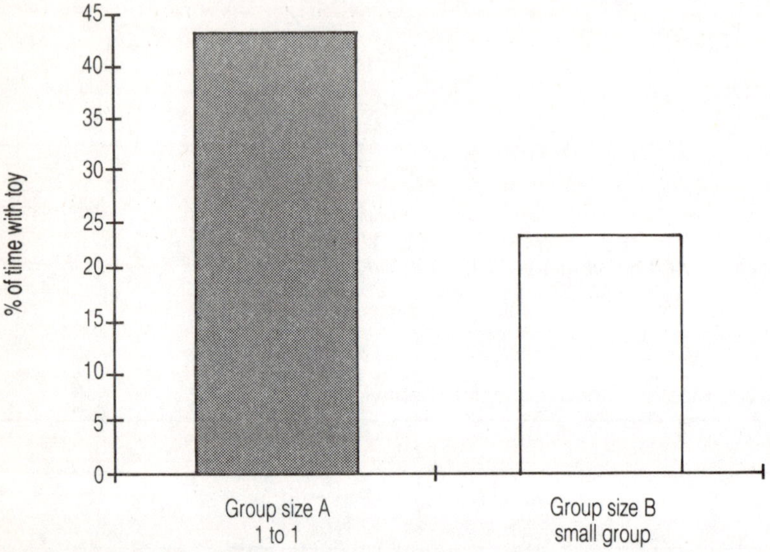

Figure 3-2: Group size and rates of possession of toy.

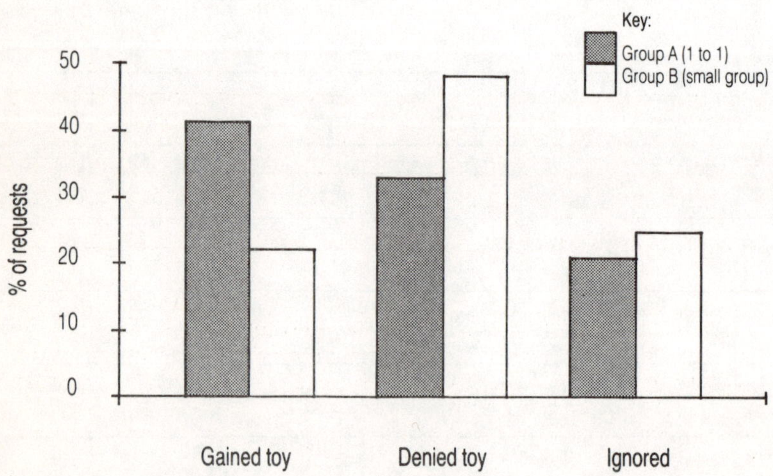

Figure 3-3: Outcomes of requests and group size.

ignored (22%:27%). The subjects were clearly more successful in requesting in the one-to-one context.

Strategies used to gain the listener's attention, gesture and body orientation were found to be moderately affected by the size of the group (see Tables 3-5, 3-6 and 3-7).

It can be seen from Table 3-5 that children tended to use the verbal/physical strategy more often in the one-to-one situation, and purely physical strategies more frequently in the larger group situation.

It can be seen from Table 3-6 that subjects were more likely to take the toy in the one-to-one situation, and more likely to reach toward the toy in the larger group situation. Instances of touching or pulling the toy were similar across both group contexts. As suggested in Table 3-7, the subjects were more likely to lean forward (toward the child with the toy) when playing in the larger group situation and more likely to stand in an erect position in the one-to-one play group. This finding is in contrast to the effect of group size on other behaviours where the small group situation tended to elicit more assertive or sophisticated behaviours.

The size of the group had very little effect on the number of requests made (164 requests in the one-to-one group compared with

Table 3-5: Group size and strategies used in requesting behaviours.

Group size	Verbal/physical %	Physical %	Other %
A (1 to 1)	53.5	33	13.5
B (small group)	41	41.5	17.5

Table 3-6: Group size and the use of gestures to request objects.

Group size	Touch/pull toy %	Take toy %	Reach for toy %	Other %
A (1 to 1)	32	35	17	16
B (small group)	33	37	24	26

Table 3-7: Group size and body orientation when requesting.

Group size	Inclined forward %	Erect %	Other %
A (1 to 1)	48.5	37.5	14
B (small group)	68.5	24.5	7

176 in the larger group), the form of the requests, voice pitch, voice volume, direction of movement, direction of gaze and facial expression (see Table 3-8).

Effects of Developmental Level

Major differences existed between the normal and the delayed groups in the amount of time the children had possession of the toy and the outcomes of their requests. The normal group had possession of the toy for a far higher percentage of the time (46% : 20% — see Figure 3-4) and were far more successful in the outcomes of their requests (46% : 21% — see Figure 3-5). However, there were found to be marked differences between individuals within both the delayed group and the normal group, in the outcomes of their requests (see Figure 3-6).

Marked differences were also demonstrated between developmental levels with regard to the gestures used. The normal group was more than twice as likely to take the toy from another child than was the delayed group (35% : 15%). The delayed group touched or pulled the toy toward them slightly more often than did the normal group (35% : 30%). The normal group did not use pointing to request at all.

Table 3-8: Group size and other forms of requesting behaviours.

Feature	Behaviour				
Direction of movement:	Toward self	Static		Other	Total
Group A (%)	54.5	39.5		6	100
Group B (%)	54	40.5		5.5	100
Direction of gaze:	Toward toy			Other	Total
Group A (%)	70			30	100
Group B (%)	64			36	100
Form:	Question	Imperative	Declarative	Other	Total
Group A (%)	30.5	26.5	16.5	26.5	100
Group B (%)	31.5	23	16.5	29	100
Facial expression:	Neutral	Smile		Other	Total
Group A (%)	50.5	18		31.5	100
Group B (%)	51	20.5		28.5	100
Voice volume:	Moderate			Other	Total
Group A (%)	86			14	100
Group B (%)	69			31	100
Voice pitch:	Moderate			Other	Total
Group A (%)	88			12	100
Group B (%)	80			20	100

Group A = 1 to 1; Group B = small group.

Instances of the use of extraneous "other" gestures and the absence of any gestures were twice as frequent in the delayed group than in the normal group (12% : 6%).

Noteworthy differences between the normal and delayed groups were also observed with regard to the direction of the subject's movement during requesting. The normal group overwhelmingly either moved toward the subject and toy or made no significant movement (99.5%). Although these were also the two most frequent movement categories used by the delayed group (89%), they moved toward and then away from the toy more frequently than the normal

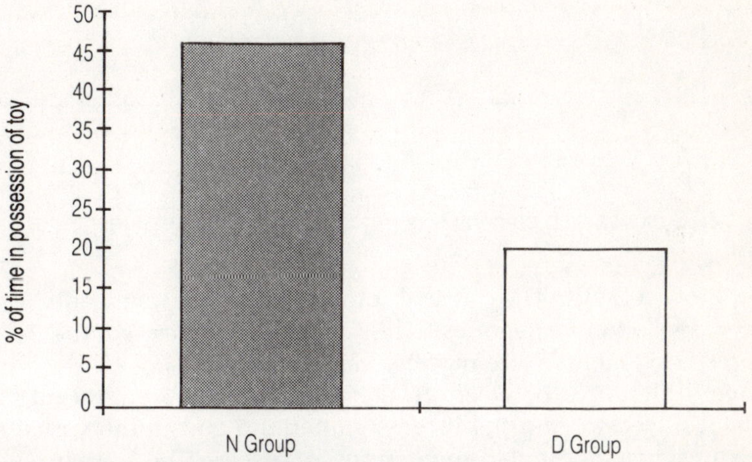

Figure 3-4: Possession of toy by each group.

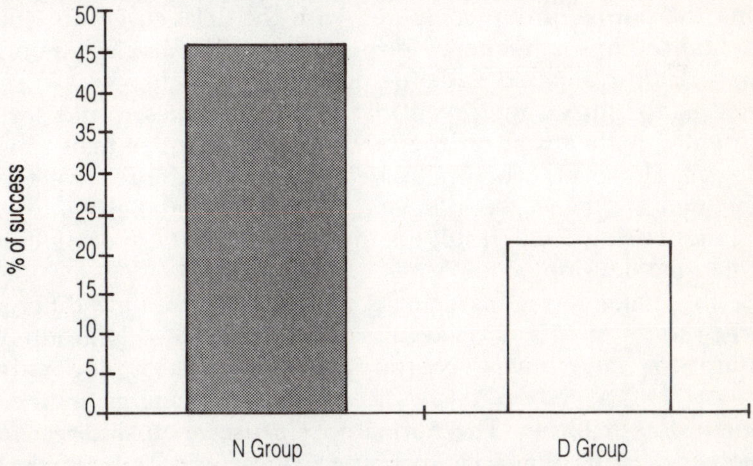

Figure 3-5: Outcomes of requests for toy for each group.

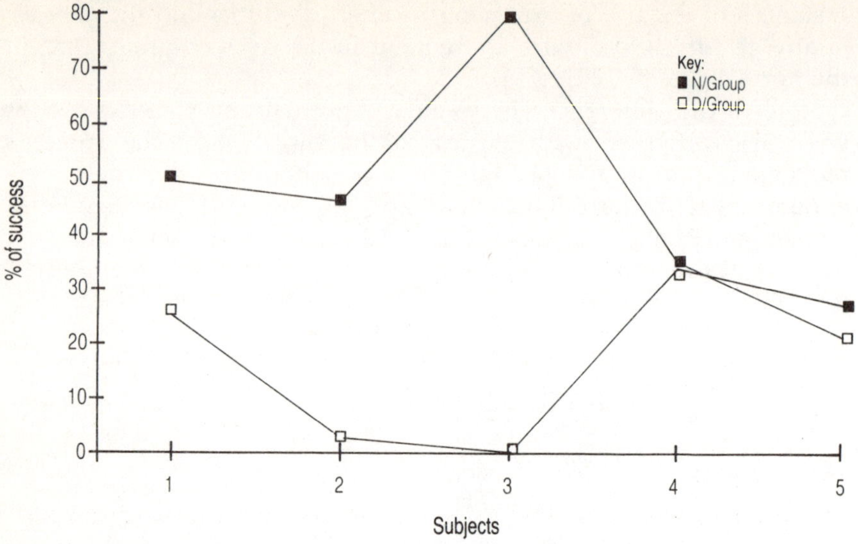

Figure 3-6: Success with outcomes of requests for individual students.

group (5% : 0.5%). The normal group had no movements in the "away" or "other" categories, while a small percentage of the delayed group's movements were in these categories (5.5%).

Some differences between developmental levels were found in the strategies used to gain the listener's attention and in the verbal form of request used. Similar frequencies of use of the verbal/physical combination were found between the two groups (normal 48% : delayed 46.5%). The higher frequency of purely physical strategies among the normal group compared with the delayed group (40.5% : 34%) and the lower frequency of purely verbal strategies among the normal group compared with the delayed group (16.5% : 9%) seems at first glance surprising, given that verbal strategies would seem to represent a higher rung in the developmental ladder than physical strategies. However, when perceived in terms of the relative success of the two strategies (see "Relationships between Behaviours and Outcomes" below), this result fits the emerging pattern of differences between the developmental levels.

For the major forms of requests used there were few differences between the normal and delayed groups (question — N group 32% : D group 33%; imperative — N group 21% : D group 24%; declarative — N group 14% : D group 19%). The differences emerge in the less frequently used forms. The normal group used both indirect forms and other verbalisation accompanying requests more frequently than the delayed group (indirect — 16% : 4%; other verbalisation —

6% : 3%). A single word to request was far more frequently used by the delayed group (11% : 5%).

The number of requests made, voice pitch, voice volume, body orientation, direction of gaze and facial expression were all found to be affected either to a small extent or not at all by developmental level.

Relationships between Behaviours and Outcomes

Strategies, gestures, verbal forms of request and direction of gaze were analysed in terms of outcomes, to identify the most successful behaviours and to determine whether noteworthy differences existed between developmental levels. The most successful strategy was found to be the verbal/physical combination, which was more successful for the normal group (N group 67% success : D group 51% success). The delayed group experienced some success with purely physical strategies. Verbal strategies used alone were unsuccessful for both groups. These results indicate the importance of physical movement and gesture for effective requesting in the preschool population.

Taking the toy was the most successful strategy for both normal and delayed subjects. It proved to be enormously successful for the normal group, who never failed when they attempted to take a toy directly from another child. Taking accounted for 71% of all successful requests in the normal group, and for 48% of all successes in the delayed group. The delayed group encountered some failure (5% denial of toy) but were never ignored when using the taking strategy.

Touching or pulling the toy was a relatively successful gesture for gaining the toy for the delayed group, accounting for 43% of successes in the delayed group and 24% of successes in the normal group. Neither the normal nor the delayed group experienced much success with reaching, touching the child or refraining from use of gesture altogether. It is interesting to note that reaching, although an unsuccessful strategy, was quite commonly used by both groups (N group 20% : D group 22%), and that refraining from any gesture, also unsuccessful, was much more commonly used by the delayed group (16% : 8%).

Failures outnumbered successes for both groups when using the imperative and declarative forms of requesting. The imperative accounted for 28% of successes and 31% of failures in the normal group, and 29% of successes and 32% of failures in the delayed group; while the declarative accounted for 15% of successes and 17.5% of failures in the normal group, and 21% of successes and 22% of failures in the delayed group. The delayed group experienced some success using the question form, which accounted for 50% of successful outcomes and 70% of all failures for this group. The use of a question was less successful for the normal group, for whom this form accounted for 24% of successes and 76% of failures. No member of the delayed group was successful at gaining the toy even once using other verbalisations or indirect forms, while for the normal group, other verbalisations and indirect forms accounted for 16.5% of successes and 18% of failures.

When looking at the child or toy, the normal group was more often successful and the delayed group more often failed. Looking away behaviours jeopardised the outcome for the normal group more often than the delayed group. These results suggests that, for the delayed group, other combinations of behaviours might be more significant in determining the outcome than direction of gaze.

Summary of Results

In general, the delayed group showed a tendency toward less mature and less effective behaviours than the normal group. Although it was not true for every behaviour, it appeared that the larger group size often elicited less mature behaviours than did the one-to-one play situation. Similarly, more sophisticated behaviours and vocalisations, such as indirect verbal forms, were evident in the one-to-one context.

Definite patterns emerged with regard to the most frequently used behaviours, possession of the toy and outcomes in relation to group size and developmental level, and the most effective behaviours for success in gaining the toy.

Discussion

The emphasis in the following section is on the relevance of the findings from the current study to the development of communication skills in children with mild developmental delay who attend preschool centres. In this discussion, requesting behaviours of normal and delayed subjects are compared, and the effect of group size on behaviours and outcomes is examined. The findings of this study are considered with regard to achieving goals of communication, the development of the request function, factors involved in successful communication, and the question of whether differences in the development of pragmatic skills in children with developmental delay constitute a qualitative difference or merely quantitative delay. Implications for preschool programs of the sociolinguistic approach to language learning are considered. Also included are the implications of the findings for the development of effective intervention programs for use in the mainstream preschool environment. Some suggestions for further studies are provided.

Requesting Behaviours of Normal and Developmentally Delayed Subjects

An aim of the current study was to investigate behaviours used to request a toy. A typical request made by the children in this study would probably have featured the use of the verbal/physical combination strategy, although nonverbal strategies were also used. The request would probably have been phrased in the form of a question, and a moderate pitch and volume of voice would have been used. The requester would probably have simply taken the toy from another child, or touched the toy or pulled it toward him or herself. He or she would probably have moved toward the child with the toy but could have remained reasonably still. A forward body orientation would have been the most likely position, although an erect posture was also observed. The subject would probably have looked toward the toy with a neutral facial expression. While there were many exceptions to this collection of behaviours associated with requesting, these were the most commonly found in the 340 requests observed.

The present study was also concerned with the differences between normal and developmentally delayed children in their requesting behaviour. It is interesting to note that the above behaviour patterns were similar for both the delayed and normal groups, with a few notable exceptions. While the normal group took the toy most often, the delayed group touched or pulled the toy most often. The next most common gesture used by the delayed group was reaching, which was found to be an unsuccessful strategy. The action of taking the toy was only the fourth most common gesture used by the delayed group. Thus, one of the most significant behaviour differences between the developmental levels was in their use of gesture.

The delayed group was relatively ineffective in its use of gesture to request a toy. While the patterns for direction of movement and body orientation were similar for both developmental levels, the delayed group showed relatively less of the forward and toward behaviours and more of the static and erect behaviours than did the normal group. It would seem that taking is a more assertive action than touching or pulling the toy, and reaching is a less assertive action still. Similarly, movements and body orientations that are toward and forward would seem to be more assertive than static positions and erect postures.

These findings appear to point to a lack of assertiveness in the behaviour of the delayed group, which may account for the children's comparative failure to achieve their goals in requesting. It also leads to speculation as to whether this lack of assertiveness is the result of previous failures causing diffidence, or the result of failure to learn the subtle factors relating to the amount of forcefulness necessary to achieve their goals. It is possible that the delayed children have not adjusted as quickly as the normal children to the slightly different behaviours required to achieve their goals when communicating with adults and peers. When communicating with caregivers, it may be possible to gain a toy by simply touching it or reaching towards it. Communication with peers seems to require a more direct approach.

The observers gained the distinct impression that, with the exception of one subject, the delayed children held a lower status in the groups than any of the normal children. It is a matter for speculation as to whether the general lack of assertiveness is the cause or result of this perceived low status. An interesting subject for a future study would be to investigate the question of the status of delayed preschoolers, and to probe its causes and results.

A striking difference between the members of the normal group and the delayed group was in the variety of their speech. The normal group's verbal output was categorised by a rich variety of forms and of actual words spoken. In contrast, three of the four delayed subjects who did use the request function showed a tendency toward repeating the same forms and even the same words constantly, even if they proved unsuccessful. An exception was the most competent communicator among the delayed group, who used many questions but also a wider variety of words and a mixture of forms.

It appears that the delayed children tended to have fewer verbal strategies at their disposal and less ability to change verbal content when the previous verbal strategies had been unsuccessful. This observation has implications for intervention programs for these children.

Effect of Play Group Size on Behaviours and Outcomes

Beveridge et al (1988) and Guralnick and Groom (1985) maintain that the success of delayed children's communications is affected by the situation in which they occur. Guralnick and Groom state that delayed children's social interactions may be influenced by: (1) the play activity the child is engaged in; (2) who the child is interacting with; (3) the types of toys involved; and (4) the extent to which teachers adopt a directive role. The findings of the current study certainly support the influence of at least the second factor, but the influence of these factors does not appear to be confined to delayed children. It was found that both delayed and normal children's interactions were influenced by both the group size and the characteristics of the children they were playing with, although the groups did not always react the same way to these factors. Further research could be conducted to determine what effect these factors have on delayed and normal children's communications.

It is interesting to note that group size affected some behaviours more than others. It particularly affected the use of strategies to gain the listener's attention, gesture and body orientation. Group size appeared to affect these behaviours in different ways. There was a tendency to use a more mature strategy (verbal/physical) than the less mature strategy (physical) in the one-to-one situation. Children tended to use more assertive gestures in the one-to-one situation. However, this pattern of the more mature, assertive and successful behaviours occurring in the one-to-one situation was reversed for body orientation. In this case, forward postures were more common in the larger group context. It is possible that the factor of body orientation is less vital in the one-to-one situation, where the child can rely on other behaviours to be noticed, while in a larger group the child may need to demonstrate intent more clearly through gross body positioning.

According to Dreyer (1987), pragmatics entails speaking politely, taking turns, defusing conflict and gaining personal goals. It has been observed that not only did the children find it easier both to be noticed and to succeed in achieving their goals in the one-to-one situation, but they were also better able to take turns with the toy in that group context. A behaviour that could be interpreted as a strategy to defuse conflict, the act of smiling, was seen much more often in the one-to-one play situation in the normal group. It appears that the pragmatic aspects of language described by Dreyer are more easily mastered in a one-to-one play situation than in a larger group. It would seem feasible, then, to begin to teach these elements to delayed children in a smaller group context and gradually to proceed to a larger group.

Pragmatics refers to the use of language in the social context. Although the group size represented only a minor change in context, it was found to have a material effect on behaviours and outcomes for the children in this study. This finding would appear to illustrate Bates' (1976b) contention that context does not just cause language but is also an integral part of language structure. Language emanated from both contexts, but the pragmatic features of the language were changed by a minor change in context.

Achieving Goals of Communication

The findings of the present study indicate that preschool children are not yet adept at achieving their requesting goals with peers. Both developmental levels had higher failure than success rates. It has already been observed that some children are much more competent at achieving their personal goals than others, and that the delayed children had more difficulty with this than the normal group. The failure rate was so high for the delayed subjects that this writer was amazed they persevered. One wonders whether these children will continue to try as they get older if they continue to meet with failure. This difficulty has implications for intervention programs, particularly for those children who will be mainstreamed at school.

An interesting observation was that often when the delayed children acquired the toy, they either were not permitted by other children or chose not to play with it for as long as the normal children did. Thus, even when the children seemed to have achieved their goal, they were in fact less successful. This observation has implications for preschool programs. If toys are in short supply, the delayed children may be less likely to have their fair share of time with the toys, thus restricting their experience in terms of having time to experiment.

An unexpected result was that, of the delayed group, the subject with the lowest measured IQ was the most successful at achieving his goals. Conversely, the subject with the highest IQ measurement did not make any requests and failed to assert herself in any way, remaining an almost totally passive onlooker. There are several possible conclusions that can be drawn from these findings. It is possible that the IQ measurements are invalid or unreliable for some reason, or that these findings may simply reflect individual differences in this very small sample of subjects. However, it is also possible that success at achieving personal goals for these children in this particular situation is not a function of intelligence.

Another similar paradox can be seen by comparing the language ability of two delayed subjects. The first had the most advanced expressive verbal language skills of the delayed group. In contrast, the other child experienced major difficulties in expressive language. Despite these language deficits, the latter child was much more successful at achieving his goals than the former. A conclusion that could be tentatively drawn from these findings is that success in requesting from peers is not necessarily a function of semantic and grammatical language abilities but may be more dependent on pragmatic aspects of language. More research with a larger sample of subjects needs to be undertaken to confirm these possibilities. If the above conclusions are confirmed, there are important implications for language intervention programs.

Implications of the Sociolinguistic Approach to Language Learning

The sociolinguistic approach emphasises reciprocity between communicators. The behaviour of the listener obviously affects the outcome for the communicator. Thus successful communication is dependent upon the behaviours of both communicator and responder. The implications of this for intervention programs are that we must teach not only communicator behaviours but also listener and respondent behaviours across many different contexts.

The sociolinguistic approach also asserts that the need to communicate effectively is the primary motivation for language learning. This was borne out in all except one of the subjects. The children were highly motivated to be effective in their communication, as it was only by communicating that they could acquire the toy that they wanted. This strengthens the argument for language learning to take place in naturally occurring settings with naturally occurring reinforcers.

In a similar vein, Norris and Hoffman (1980) maintain that children discover properties of language through immersion in the communicative process. It can be seen from the observations that learning was going on throughout. Children, especially those in the normal group, were changing strategies when they learned that previous behaviours were not successful. An example of this from the transcript of an observation of a subject from the normal group in a larger play group was as follows:

"Can I have a go?"
"It's my go now."
"Can I've a go now, Megan? . . . Megan?"
"I'm going after you, aren't I?"

This child was trying out new request forms and strategies. She was not only finding out the effectiveness of these strategies but also practising different modes of making the same request.

Sequence of Development of the Request Function

Owens (1988) suggested a sequence of development of requesting beginning with: (1) gesture; (2) gesture plus vocalisation; (3) gaze toward partner, two coordinated gestures in sequence or gesture plus conventional word. The stage three constellation of behaviours comprising gaze toward partner and gesture plus verbalisation was the most frequently seen in this study. Stage one behaviour, gesture without vocalisation, was also frequently seen but usually in conjunction with gaze toward child or toy. Gesture plus vocalisation was rarely seen in either group.

It is interesting that the delayed group used stage three behaviours much more frequently in the one-to-one context, and stage one behaviours much more frequently in the larger group context. It may be that these children felt more at ease in the one-to-one situation, where they were more successful, and were consequently able to use more sophisticated strategies than they could in the larger group.

Wood (1981) maintains that gesture becomes less critical as children become more verbal and that preschool children still rely heavily on gesture to convey their message. The findings of the current study concur with the suggestion that preschool children rely heavily on gesture. The fact that gesture is still critical is borne out by the low frequency of purely verbal strategies and the high failure rate when those strategies were in operation. The fact that some gestures were strongly associated with success points to the continuing importance of gesture for this age group.

Moerk (1977) proposed three stages of gesture/verbal combinations in the development of referring to specific objects and events: (1) parallel encoding (simultaneous use of words and gesture, with heavy reliance on gesture and incidental use of words); (2) verbal complementation (rather ambiguous gesture, clarified by verbal message); (3) substitution of verbal forms (most information carried verbally, with gesture somewhat redundant). The results of the present study suggest that, for the request function, most of the subjects appeared to be at the parallel-encoding stage, with some showing signs of the verbal complementation stage. As demonstrated in the previous paragraph, these children were not ready to substitute verbal forms for gesture when requesting a toy from a peer. That is not to say that these same subjects would not be at a more advanced stage when using a different pragmatic function, with a different listening audience.

Surprisingly, the delayed group used purely verbal strategies more often than the normal group. These strategies were not successful in terms of outcome for either group. As these strategies may be successful with an adult communicative partner, the question of adaptation to the characteristics of the listener is again raised. Do the delayed children have more difficulty than the normal children in adjusting to the requirements of a peer as a communicative partner rather than an adult?

Garvey (1975) divided verbal requests into three forms: (1) direct (for example, "Gimme that truck."); (2) indirect (such as "Will you give me that truck?"); and (3) inferred. Garvey's inferred request corresponds to what is termed indirect in the current study (such as "I can make a tunnel too," said while pulling the toy toward himself). Garvey found that preschoolers used the direct (imperative) form most often but it was only 53% successful. This form was the second most frequently used by the subjects in the current study, accounting for 28.5% of all successes and carrying a 48% success rate. Garvey found that her indirect form (a question) was used far less often but had a 75% success rate. In contrast, the subjects in this study used questions the most often. Questions accounted for 37% of all successes and carried a 50% success rate. This writer does not have information on whether the communicative partners of the children in Garvey's study were adults or children. This would affect the success rate.

Bates (1971, quoted in Bates, 1976a) found that almost all requests by the preschool children in her study were either imperatives or declaratives. The results of the current study showed that questions, imperatives and declaratives, in that order, accounted for most of the requests. Owens (1988) stated that five-year-olds can make some inferred requests, although this was most infrequent. The subjects in the present study, ranging in age from four and a half to five and a half years, made inferred requests 6.75% of the time, with this form being far more prevalent in the normal group. Findings from the current study support Owens and all the other researchers who maintain that forms of requesting move from direct to indirect, explicit to less explicit, and simple to complex.

Factors Involved in Successful Communication

Previous research has found that such nonverbal factors as eye contact, gesture, facial expression, body position and moving closer to the listener were important in gaining and maintaining the attention of the listener (Kendon & Cook, 1979; Lucas, 1980; Mueller, 1972; Ochs & Schieffelin, 1983). Nonverbal behaviours, especially gesture, were found to be significant in terms of outcome for the current subjects. Most delayed children used appropriate eye contact, and inappropriate eye contact did not appear to have a substantial effect on outcome for the delayed group in this study. Facial expression tended to be relatively uniform among all subjects, so was not considered to be crucial toward the outcome. Body position and direction of movement and their relationship to outcome was not investigated in this study due to lack of time. Because the normal group was more successful and tended to adopt forward body orientations and movements more often than the delayed group, one would expect that these two factors would be associated with success.

In agreement with Mueller (1972), it was found that the lack of attention-getting techniques was a powerful predictor of failure. For example, when children failed to use gesture or to look in the direction of the toy or child, they were more likely to fail. Mueller maintained that some verbal or vocal form of securing the listener's attention, combined with nonverbal techniques, was crucial to success. As has been mentioned earlier, this combination was also found to be the most successful in the current study.

Wood (1981) stated that agreement of body language with verbal language was crucial to success. This would appear to have been the case with the current subjects. The most unsuccessful requester used quite sophisticated verbal language but often failed to complement it with nonverbal cues such as gesture, gaze, body position and movement to convey her message. The consensus of opinion from former studies is that success or failure is not attributable to a single behaviour but to a whole range of verbal and nonverbal behaviours, acting in harmony with the function. The findings of the present study support this contention.

Pragmatic Skills in Children with Developmental Delay: Delay or Difference?

The matter of whether delayed children use normal pragmatic skills was a question of debate in previous studies, with conflicting results. In the current study, the subjects were too few for the findings to suggest a valid conclusion. However, the results from this study were conflicting as well. The delayed group as a whole did tend to be less effective communicators than the normal group. They also talked less and played a less dominant role as a group than the normal group, a finding shared by Kamhi and Masterson (1988). They were more inclined to use fewer words or no words than the normal group.

In contrast with the results of Snyder (1975), this study did not find that the delayed children had difficulty expressing imperative and declarative forms. The findings of the present study did mirror Oller et al's (1978) findings, that normal children used more sophisticated strategies, such as indirect requests, more than did the delayed children. Cooper (1986) found a difference between the developmental levels in the types of directives used with the normal group using questions and the delayed group tending to use short, repetitive imperatives. Although members of the delayed group in the current study were inclined to use shorter utterances and to be more repetitive, there was no substantial difference in their use of questions, imperatives and declaratives.

Despite the tendency for the delayed group to be less effective communicators, one subject was as effective as his normal matched partner. This child's pragmatic skills seem to be similar to those of normal children despite his lower IQ and his language delay. In contrast, another delayed subject appeared to have quite a different pattern of development relating to pragmatic skills, as her communications did not merely reflect immature development but demonstrated abnormal patterns. Examples of this are the prevalence of unusual and extraneous hand movements and frequently no gestures at all; a significantly higher proportion than the other children of meaningless and ineffective movements and body positions; and frequent instances of gaze away from the toy and child. This child also appeared to have little awareness of the effect of her behaviour on others. Another subject could make no requests to her peers. Her difficulty with the pragmatic aspects of language is obvious despite her relatively good command of the semantic and grammatical aspects of language. Two subjects showed an immature rather than a substantially different pattern from that of the normal group.

Concerning the question of delay or difference in the pragmatic language of delayed children, Prutting and Kirchner (1983) suggested three possible subgroups of delayed children who have the following problems:

1. Social — children lacking sensitivity to various dimensions of the social context
2. Cognitive — children for whom a cognitive deficit places a limit on potential for communicative competence
3. Linguistic — children who have difficulties with high-level linguistic operations.

Each of the delayed children in the current study who demonstrated deficits in communication could possibly be identified as belonging to one of the above subgroups. However, these distinctions would be arbitrary as most also showed some features of other subgroups. Although these subgroups offer one feasible explanation of the contradictory evidence regarding delay or difference in the pragmatic skills of delayed children, it is the opinion of this writer that these subgroups may not be mutually exclusive and that some children may have elements of all three problems.

Fey and Leonard (1983) also found three distinct behaviour patterns, similar to those of Prutting and Kirchner. They categorised the groups according to degrees of social interaction: the first group being those unresponsive to social interaction; the second group being responsive to social partners but unassertive in interaction; and the third group corresponding to Prutting and Kirchner's third group, with no qualitative pragmatic differences but limited by difficulties of linguistic form.

While some of the delayed subjects in this study could be classified as belonging to the unassertive group, and others could be seen to be mainly limited by linguistic difficulties, these distinctions may not tell the whole story, as some characteristics of the second and third groups appeared to be common to at least three of the five children. One child did not fit into any of Fey and Leonard's categories. This writer agrees with Fey and Leonard that further investigations are needed on this subject before the theory of distinct groups based on degrees of social interaction could serve to explain adequately the conflicting findings regarding qualitative versus quantitative differences, or to aid the practitioner in the development of intervention programs.

Implications for Intervention Programs

The current study showed that the delayed children were not as effective as a group at achieving their personal requesting goals as the normal children were. The ability or inability to achieve one's goals through communication with others appears to affect one's quality of life fundamentally. Continued failure may also depress motivation to continue to communicate with peers. Intervention programs must therefore provide children with the skills and behaviours that will allow them to be successful communicators with their normal peers in mainstream environments.

Prutting and Kirchner's and Fey and Leonard's work of identifying subgroups of pragmatic language deficit and the variation in behaviours of the delayed group in the current study demonstrate that the simple identification of a specific deficit in the pragmatic area (such as the request function) is not sufficient information on which to base an intervention program for an individual child. The evidence from this study also demonstrates that the practitioner should not assume communicative competence to be necessarily related to IQ levels or to the form and content of language for the mildly delayed population. Instead, the teacher would be advised to observe carefully each child's behaviours and outcomes in communication with peers, before making any decisions regarding communicative competence or intervention programs. For the specific needs of the delayed communicator to be met, it is necessary to isolate points of strength and identify areas of difficulty before embarking on any intervention program.

As effective communication appears to be attributable not simply to one behaviour but to a range of behaviours, nonverbal behaviours such as gesture, eye contact, body positioning as well as verbal behaviours need to be observed. It is important for the practitioner to consider such questions as:

Are all behaviours congruent with the function of the communication?

Are the communicative behaviours appropriate for the developmental stage of the listener?

Are the behaviours appropriate for the specific communicative context (such as a language group led by the teacher versus an unstructured play situation)?

If impediments to successful communication are isolated through this process, then effective behaviours need to be specifically taught across a wide range of contexts. It may be necessary to teach specific communicative behaviours appropriate for particular contexts, as many delayed children appear to have difficulties "reading" subtle differences in social context and adjusting their behaviour accordingly. The intervention program may also include the elimination of behaviours that detract from effective communication, such as extraneous hand movements or other distracting body language.

The fact that immersion in the communicative process provides motivation for language learning is a reason for intervention to take place in natural play settings, which are meaningful to the child, instead of in isolated clinical settings. Another implication is that programs should provide for naturally occurring reinforcers rather than those that are artificially contrived. Achieving a communicative goal is an intrinsic reinforcer of behaviour.

If language is learned through immersion in the communication process, then the development of effective communication with peers must be facilitated by arranging opportunities for the delayed child to have as much interaction as possible with peers in as many situations as possible. Simply allowing delayed children to be in the same location as their non-delayed peers does not necessarily mean that communicative interaction will take place. The teacher may need to facilitate the interaction at first by helping the child join the group, modelling appropriate behaviours and "repairing" communications initially to smooth the communication path.

Built into the intervention program should be the gradual withdrawal of adult support. Too often in mainstream settings, adults continue to provide support when the delayed child is ready to move toward more independence in their interactions. This fosters adult dependence and "learned helplessness".

It is possible that opportunities for constant active participation in communicative play situations with peers is even more important for delayed children than for their normal peers. Too often practitioners train delayed children to communicate with adults and assume that these skills will automatically be transferred to the much more difficult task of communicating with peers. As children with developmental delay cannot transfer skills across contexts as readily as their non-delayed peers, this method of teaching children to communicate would seem to be ineffective.

Communication with peers is more difficult as children do not interpret and "repair" conversations as adults do. In the opinion of this writer, children with developmental delay often require both specific training in particular communicative behaviours and the opportunity, through frequent supervised practice, to develop a "feeling" for the constellation of behaviours that will be successful with a given listener.

As a minor change in context was shown to affect behaviours and outcomes of requests quite significantly, one must look carefully at the situation in which the communications are taking place before deciding on a course of intervention. It is important to identify situational factors that present difficulties for a particular child, such as structured or unstructured conditions, the gender and age of communicative partners, the presence or absence of adults, so that the child can be specifically trained to cope with the communicative demands of these situations.

The subjects in the current study were more often able to use relatively more sophisticated and assertive behaviours, achieved more communicative success and were more likely to gain opportunities to play with a desired toy in the one-to-one situation with another child. Because the delayed child may have a more successful experience in terms of getting to play with a toy and of others responding to his requests in the one-to-one situation, this context would provide greater motivation for the initial development of requesting behaviours.

Similarly, in the one-to-one context the child would gain more practice in the use of the more successful behaviours such as the verbal/physical form of attention-getting and assertive gestures. It would seem logical, then, for new behaviours to be practised in a one-to-one situation, before gradually progressing to larger groups.

Intervention programs should aim for appropriate interaction with peers in all commonly occurring situations. It is particularly important that preschool children gain skills in playground interactions. Integration support in infant and primary (or elementary) schools is often concentrated in the classroom and aimed primarily at academic progress. Thus mildly delayed children are often unsupported in unstructured out-of-classroom school activities. It can be argued that these situations more closely reflect "real life" and hold important implications for successful peer interaction during out-of-school time and for future social acceptance. Some examples of the kinds of skills required are: strategies for joining a group; sharing equipment; requesting a turn; and following rules of games.

After assessing needs and examining the context, one would aim to teach more sophisticated and successful strategies than those currently being employed. For the particular group of delayed subjects in this study, it would be appropriate to model and encourage the use of more verbal/physical combination strategies. One method of achieving this is to structure a one-to-one play situation with a desired toy, using a peer who is an effective communicator as a role model. The adult can prompt the delayed child to imitate appropriate verbal and nonverbal behaviours used by the other child. The child can graduate to structured small group situations once the behaviours have been mastered in the one-to-one context.

The importance of effective nonverbal strategies has been demonstrated. Nonverbal behaviours such as appropriate gaze, gesture, movement and body orientation in relation to the listener could be modelled and practised. The delayed group in the current study appeared to use ineffective gestures. Structured role-playing and miming games that are designed to achieve a communicative goal could be helpful if the teacher ensured that the outcome of each game directly related to the appropriateness of the gesture used. Skills learned in these structured situations should always be generalised in normal play situations.

Congruence of body language with verbal output and pragmatic function may need to be systematically taught in many different situations. Behaviours such as coming close to the listener in order to be seen and heard, facing the listener, looking at the listener, calling his or her name and using an appropriate gesture are learned incidentally by most children but often need to be specifically learned and practised by children with deficits in the pragmatic area of language.

An intervention program should also take into account the need for awareness of the listener's response and for the ability to change behaviour accordingly. This implies both monitoring the communicative partner's behaviour and possessing a repertoire of strategies so that a change in technique is possible.

In order to equip children to change strategies according to listener response, they should be exposed to and practise a variety of verbal and nonverbal forms to achieve the same end. It may be important to teach delayed children to use imperatives, declaratives and questions and to practise their use in a variety of situations. They may need to be encouraged to switch forms when their first attempt is unsuccessful. The methods of modelling, imitation and practice can be used. A possible teaching sequence could begin with the use of puppets while interacting with one adult, with the adult structuring the game to require the child to alter the request form before the puppet complies with the request. The use of puppets often lends humour to the situation and gives confidence to the child. The activity could then be implemented with or without puppets in one-to-one situations with another child, and finally in small groups across many contexts.

The development of a repertoire of suitable words and phrases for requesting can be encouraged by working in small groups that include competent communicators. Asking the group such questions as "What is another way we can ask for the car?" and letting them practise their suggestions could provide a valuable learning experience.

Children can be helped to become conscious of the effect of their behaviour on others. They can be trained to look for and expect a response and to modify their behaviour accordingly. For example, when a child's communication has not gained a response, the adult could say, "Look at Mary. Did she hear you?" The adult could then suggest that the child call the listener and/or tap her on the shoulder and perhaps could model words or actions for the child to imitate.

Awareness of the communicative partner also includes knowing the different demands placed upon the communicator by communicative partners of different ages. For example, some behaviours may be effective and appropriate when communicating with adults, but other behaviours may be required when communicating with peers.

To help children become more aware of listener response and the need to change behaviour accordingly, an adult could initially play the role of the listener while the children try various requesting strategies. The adult could structure play situations where perhaps more assertive actions or more polite forms of request are necessary to achieve goals. This could be followed by supported practice in the natural play environment, with the adult providing prompts as necessary, and the gradual phasing out of adult support.

Although no data were collected on the timing of requests, it was noted from the observations that waiting for the right moment to request seemed to play an important part in the success of requests. The children who successfully used the taking gesture accompanied by a verbal request tended to wait for an appropriate time while another child had a turn. When the toy ran down or at some other natural break in the play, these children made their request. In contrast, the delayed children often seemed to lack that sense of timing. They sometimes requested the toy immediately and constantly and were often simply ignored. This indicates that children should be made aware of the need to wait for the appropriate moment.

It may be helpful for an adult to stop the child from making an immediate request by saying something like "Wait for Peter to finish his turn" and then, at the opportune moment, prompting him by saying "Now ask for a turn". With frequent practice, the child may begin to develop his own sense of timing in order to maximise the success of requesting goals.

In addition to becoming communicators, delayed children need to learn the appropriate behaviours of a listener and respondent. As interactions require reciprocity and the success of a communication is largely dependent on the reaction of the listener, responding behaviours are of great importance to ongoing, effective communications.

Another factor of importance to intervention programs is the high failure rate in achieving requesting goals, particularly for the delayed subjects. This can be partially addressed by learning communicative skills, but it is also important for the child to experience success frequently at his or her current level of skill.

One method of promoting successful experiences is to structure the preschool or child care centre into family-type groupings with a mix of preschool age groups, for part of the day. This would allow the delayed child to interact with children who are at a similar or earlier stage of development and give opportunities for more successful experiences, particularly in the area of requesting. Adults may also arrange opportunities for the child with mild developmental delay to model appropriate requesting behaviours for younger children, thus reinforcing the behaviours and promoting self-esteem. Achieving success in communication with peers is crucial, as the child may either give up on communication with peers or resort to inappropriate behaviour if he or she faces constant failure. The communication factor needs to be monitored as the child progresses into the mainstream school environment.

The children who are most at risk of avoiding social interaction are those who do not have the basic pragmatic functions, such as requesting from peers, in their repertoire. For these children, an intervention program should address several issues. Firstly, the program should provide motivation to request. The teacher would need to observe a child closely to ascertain which activities or conditions would successfully motivate him or her to request. Secondly, the program must provide a safe environment in which to request. This would also vary from child to child, but might include such factors as a cooperative child as a communicative partner and initial adult support. Thirdly, the program should teach behaviours that would enable the child to be successful and finally foster independence in interactions with peers.

It might be necessary to work with both normal and delayed children to raise the status of the delayed children in the group. A first step would be to evaluate the behaviour of all adults in the classroom in terms of the promotion of an atmosphere of not merely accepting but valuing individual differences such as race, language and so on. To do this, it is helpful to have one adult simply observe for a period to note which prevailing behaviours promote or detract from these values.

One of the most simple methods of raising the status of an individual within a group is to arrange for him or her to control the distribution of a desired object or activity. Observations of classrooms reveal that the children chosen for this role are often those who already enjoy high status with the children and adults, usually children who are capable and reliable. The delayed child can be given frequent opportunities to play this role, especially if adequate support is given to ensure an acceptable level of competence. This support may be provided by rehearsals before the event to teach appropriate skills and behaviours.

Teaching assertiveness techniques to the delayed children could help to raise their status and self-esteem. Apart from teaching appropriate and successful requesting behaviours, delayed children often need to be taught how to assert themselves when exposed to the aggressive behaviour of other children. Practising the art of saying "no" and defending the possession of a toy can begin with puppet play. The puppet's behaviour can be modelled by the adult first and then copied by the child. This can be followed by role-playing in simulated play situations with small groups, where nonverbal behaviours such as firmly planted feet and crossed arms accompanying the "no" can be taught, followed by initial adult support and reminders in real life situations.

Another issue that arose from the present study was that of the time a child possessed the toy. The delayed group actually got to play with the toy for a much shorter period of time than did the normal group. In view of this, preschools need to ensure that delayed children have at least equal access to opportunities for development through handling and experimenting with materials.

Even when the children with developmental delay were given opportunities to play with the toys, they often chose not to play with them for as long as the others, or tended to use them in repetitive ways. As delayed children are sometimes not as inquisitive as other preschoolers, they may need to be shown different ways of using materials and encouraged to discover new uses for themselves. In this way, productive time with materials may be prolonged and enriched.

Conclusions

It can be seen that the current study raised many issues in relation to intervention programs. The aim of intervention is to provide the delayed child with the behaviours and skills that will allow him or her to become a successful communicator, with the ability to achieve personal goals through communication. The person who implements the intervention must be cognisant of stages in the development of the request function and of individual strengths and weaknesses, as well as being familiar with the effects of the particular context on the behaviour of an individual or group.

It is desirable for intervention to take place in natural settings with naturally occurring reinforcers, and for newly learned behaviours to be initially practised in smaller group settings. The program needs to ensure opportunities for success in interactions in order to encourage children to persevere and to raise their self-esteem. The needs of children who are lacking the request function need to be addressed. Once the function is being used, one would aim toward more sophisticated strategies, the appropriate use of nonverbal behaviours and the ability to use a variety of communication forms to achieve an end.

Efforts should be made to raise the status of delayed children in the group. Training in assertiveness may be helpful to achieve this end. The program needs to include awareness of the communicative partner and the necessity to vary behaviours accordingly. Similarly, the obligations and behaviours of listening and responding need to be systematically taught to the delayed children. Delayed children need to be allowed adequate time to use play materials.

Although broad implications cannot be drawn from this study and translated into intervention programs due to the nature of the subject sample, the above suggestions would seem to be useful as general guidelines to follow for preschool children with developmental delays who have difficulty with the pragmatic aspects of language.

Suggestions for Further Studies

It can be seen that the current study leaves many questions unanswered. The findings also need to be confirmed by replication, using a large number of subjects from different preschool environments. To give a broader picture of the request function, other types of requesting could be observed in a variety of play situations — at home and at preschool, with adults, peers and siblings. A comparison of behaviours and outcomes when children are communicating with partners of different ages would be interesting. Another interesting study would be an investigation of the differences between groups of male and female preschoolers in their requesting, sharing behaviour and in group organisation. While this study was concerned only with children with mild delay, it would be interesting to study the request function in children with moderate delay, to compare their behaviours and outcomes when they communicated with peers in a special school environment, and with peers in a regular school environment. Finally, larger scale projects would lend themselves to the use of effective statistical techniques which were not available to this researcher.

Summary

The current project involved an observational study undertaken in a natural setting. The requesting behaviours of mildly developmentally delayed and non-delayed preschool children were investigated in their play with peers in two different contexts. The subjects were five developmentally delayed preschool children and five age- and sex-matched peers. All children attended mainstream preschool classes and came from three preschools in a large rural town. A trial of planned data collection procedures was conducted prior to the study. Each child was observed playing with toys on six occasions in the classroom, for approximately five minutes each time. Half of the observations were conducted while the subjects were playing with one other peer, and half were conducted in a group situation with three to four children. Observations were recorded on videotape and transcribed onto raw data sheets containing checklists of behaviours derived from the findings of previous studies.

A common pattern of behaviours associated with requesting was found to exist. Group size and developmental level were found to have major effects on the rate of possession of the toy and the outcomes of requests. These factors also affected some requesting behaviours. All children experienced more success in the one-to-one situation. The normal group was found to be more successful in terms of outcome than the delayed group and generally exhibited more mature behaviours. Some behaviours were found to be more significant in terms of outcome than others.

The degree to which the results of this study can be generalised is severely limited owing to the nature and size of the subject sample. However, the findings supported the results of previous studies on the pattern of development of requesting behaviours and on the importance of nonverbal language. The current study could add little that is definitive to the argument regarding the developmental patterns of delayed children constituting simple delay or inherent difference, as examples of both patterns were found in the results. However, members of the delayed group were shown to be less effective communicators.

The tentative conclusions drawn from, and questions raised by, the findings of this study indicate the need for undertaking further studies with large numbers of subjects from the whole environmental spectrum in many different play contexts. The relative ineffectiveness of the delayed group as communicators supports the need for intervention programs in this area. Some general suggestions for intervention programs relating to the findings of the present study have been put forward.

With the growth of our base of knowledge about the development of the pragmatic language functions of children in general, and the characteristics and needs of the delayed population in their use of these functions in particular, will come a firmer foundation on which to base intervention programs to help delayed children become more effective communicators. As language is the one ability that makes us truly human, effective communication with our peers is basic to our quality of life, and necessary for normalisation of the developmentally delayed population. It is therefore crucial that more studies are undertaken in this field of developmental pragmatics.

References

Argyle, M. (1980). Language and social interaction. In H. Giles, W.P. Robinson & P.M. Smith (eds), *Language: Social psychological perspectives*. Oxford: Pergamon Press.

Atkinson, M. (1979). Prerequisites to reference. In E. Ochs & B.B. Schieffelin (eds), *Developmental pragmatics*. New York: Academic Press.

Bates, E. (1976a). Pragmatics and sociolinguistics in child language. In D.M. Morehead & A.E. Morehead (eds), *Normal and deficient child language*. Baltimore: University Park Press.

Bates, E. (1976b). *Language and context: The acquisition of pragmatics*. New York: Academic Press.

Bates, E., Benigni, L., Bretherton, I., Camaioni, L. & Voltera, V. (1979). *The emergence of symbols: Cognition and communication in infancy*. New York: Acedemic Press.

Bernard-Opitz, V. (1982). Pragmatic analysis of the communicative behavior of an autistic child. *Journal of Speech and Hearing Disorders*, 99–109.

Bernstein, D.K. & Tiegerman, E. (1989). *Language and communication disorders in children* (2nd edn). Columbus: Charles E. Merrill.

Beveridge, M., Conti-Ramsden, G. & Leudar, I. (eds) (1988). *Language and communication in mentally handicapped people*. London: Chapman & Hall.

Bloom, L. & Lahey, M. (1978). *Language development and language disorders*. New York: John Wiley & Sons.

Bruner, J.S. (1975). The ontogenesis of speech acts. *Journal of Child Language 2*, 1–19.

Bruner, J.S. (1981). The pragmatics of acquisition. In W. Deutsch (ed.), *The child's construction of language*. London: Academic Press.

Bryen, D.N. (1981). Perspectives on the acquisition of language. In *Inquiries into child language*. Boston: Allyn & Bacon.

Campbell, R.N. & Smith, P.T. (eds) (1978). *Recent advances in the psychology of language* (111 vol. 4B). New York: Plenum Press.

Cecconi, C.P. (1987). *Intervention strategies for pragmatically impaired preschoolers: The classroom context*. New York: The Special Children's Centre.

Cirrin, F.M. & Rowland, C.M. (1985). Communicative assessment of non-verbal youths with severe/profound mental retardation. *Mental Retardation 23*, 2, 52–62.

Coggins, T.E. & Carpenter, R.L. (1980). The communicative intention inventory: A system for observing and coding children's early intentional communication. *Applied Psycholinguistics 2*, 3, 235–51.

Cooper, C.S. (1986). *A study of pragmatic skill development in two groups of young children mildly retarded and non handicapped*. Lawrence: School of Education, University of Kansas.

Corsaro, W. (1981). The development of social cognition in preschool children: Implications for language learning. *Topics in Language Disorders 1*, 77–95.

Craig, H.K. (1983). Application of pragmatic language models for intervention. In T.M. Gallagher & C.A. Prutting (eds), *Pragmatic assessment and intervention issues in language*. San Diego: College Hill Press.

Cross, T. (1977). Mothers' speech adjustments: The contribution of selected listener variables. In E.E. & C.A. Ferguson (eds), *Talking to children*. New York: Cambridge University Press.

Ditchburn, S.J. (1985). *Toward an understanding of children's play: A conversational analysis approach*. University of Calgary, Dept of Curriculum and Instruction.

Dore, J. (1975). Holophrases, speech acts and language universals. *Journal of Child Language 2*, 21–40.

Dore, J. (1977). Children's illocutionary acts. In R.O. Freedle (ed.), *Discourse production and comprehension*. Norwood: Ablex Publishing Corp.

Dore, J. (1978). Conditions for the acquisition of speech acts. In I. Markova (ed.), *The social context of language*. Chichester: John Wiley and Sons.

Dreyer, B. (1987). Pragmatics in child language: Putting language intervention into the mainstream of living. *The Pointer 32*, 29–30.

Ervin-Tripp, S. (1980). Lecture, University of Minnesota, 14 May 1980.

Fey, M.C. & Leonard, L.B. (1983). Pragmatic skills of children with specific language impairment. In T.M. Gallagher & C.A. Prutting (eds), *Pragmatic assessment and intervention issues in language*. San Diego: College Hill Press.

Field, T. (1980). Self, teacher, toy and peer directed behaviours of handicapped preschool children. In T.M. Field, S. Goldberg, D. Stern & A.M. Sostek (eds), *High risk infants and children*. New York: Academic Press.

French, L.A., Lucariello, J., Seidman, S. & Nelson, K. (1985). The influence of discourse content on preschoolers' use of language. In L. Galda & A.D. Pellegrini (eds), *Play language and stories: The development of children's literate behaviour*. Norwood: Ablex Publishing Co.

French, P. & MacLure, M. (eds) (1981). *Adult-child conversation*. London: Croom Helm.

Friel-Patti, S. & Lougeay-Mottinger, J. (1985). Preschool language intervention: Some key concerns. *Topics in Language Disorders 5 (2)*, 46–57.

Gallagher, T.M. & Prutting, C.A. (eds) (1983). *Pragmatic assessment and intervention issues in language.*, San Diego: College Hill Press.

Garvey, C. (1975). Requests and responses in child speech. *Journal of Child Language 2*, 41–63.

Garvey, C. & Hogan, R. (1988). Social speech and social interaction: Egocentrism revisited. In M.B. Franklin & S.S. Barten (eds), *Child language: A reader*. New York: Oxford University Press.

Giles, H., Robinson, W.P. & Smith, P.M. (eds) (1980). *Language: Social psychological perspectives*. Oxford: Pergamon Press.

Guralnick, M.J. & Groom, J.M. (1985). Correlates of peer-related social competence of developmentally delayed children. *American Journal of Mental Deficiency 90*, 140–50.

Halliday, M.A.K. (1975). *Learning how to mean: Explorations in the development of language*. London: Edward Arnold.

Kamhi, A.U. & Masterson, J.J. (1988). Last rites for the difference-delay controversy. In M. Beveridge, G. Conti-Ramsden & I. Leudar (eds), *Language and communication in mentally handicapped people*. London: Chapman and Hall.

Kendon, A. & Cook, M. (1979). The consistency of gaze patterns in social interaction. *British Journal of Psychology 69*, 481–94.

Klecan-Aker, J. & Lopez, E. (1984). A clinical taxonomy for the categorization of pragmatic language functions in normal preschool children. *Journal of Communication Disorders 17*, 121–31.

Leonard, L.B. (1980). The speech of language disabled children. *Bulletin of the Orton Society 30*, 141–52.

Linfoot, K.W. (1987). *Communicative behaviour in children with severe developmental delay. Unpublished doctoral dissertation*. Sydney: School of Education, Macquarie University.

Linfoot, K. & Bochner, S. (1989). *Dependent variables in research with children having developmental delay*. Paper presented to the 1989 conference of the Australian Association for Research in Education, Adelaide.

Lowell, E.L., Curtiss, S., Bennett, T.L., Prutting, C., Rouin, C. & Dunlea, A. (1977). *A search for performatives in young deaf children: A final report*. Washington, DC: US Department of Health, Education Welfare, National Institute of Education (ENC Document Reproduction Service N. EO 152048).

Lucas, E.V. (1980). *Semantic and pragmatic language disorders: Assessment and remediation*. Rockville: Aspen.

McLean, J.E. & Snyder-McLean, L.K. (1978). *A transactional approach to early language training*. Columbus: Merrill.

MacLure, M. & French, P. (1981). A comparison of talk at home and at school. In G. Wells (ed.), *Learning through interaction: The study of language development*. Cambridge: Cambridge University Press.

McShane, J. (1980). *Learning to talk*. Cambridge: Cambridge University Press.

McTear, M.F. (1979). Hey! I've got something to tell you: A study of the initiation of conversational exchanges by preschool children. *Journal of Pragmatics 3*, 321–36.

Messervy, D.M. (1990). *Communicative strategies for toy and peer directed requesting behaviours employed by normal and developmentally delayed preschool children*. Unpublished report. Bathurst: Charles Sturt University-Mitchell.

Mitchell, D.R. (1980). Down's syndrome children in structured dyadic communication situations with their parents. In J. Hogg & P. Mittler (eds), *Advances in mental handicap research*. Chichester: John Wiley & Sons.

Moerk, E.L. (1977). *Pragmatic and semantic aspects of early language development*. Baltimore: University Park Press.

Mueller, E. (1972). The maintenance of verbal exchanges between young children. *Child Development 43*, 930–48.

Newport, E., Gleitman, H. & Gleitman, L. (1977). Mother, I'd rather do it myself: Some effects and non-effects of maternal speech style. In E.E. Snow & C.A. Ferguson (eds), *Talking to children: Language input and acquisition*. New York: Cambridge University Press.

Norris, J.A. & Hoffman, P.R. (1980). Comparison of adult-initiated vs. child-initiated interaction styles with handicapped prelanguage children. *Language, Speech and Hearing Services in Schools*, 28–36.

Ochs, E. (1983). Introduction. In E. Ochs & B.B. Schieffelin (eds), *Acquiring conversational competence*. London: Routledge and Kegan Paul.

Ochs, E. & Schieffelin, B.B. (1983). *Acquiring conversational competence*. London: Routledge and Kegan Paul.

Oller, D., Thorp, T. & Coleman, D.A. (1978). *Natural logic of pragmatic function of language*. Paper presented at the Third Annual Boston Conference on Language Development.

Owens, J.E. (1988). *Language development: An Introduction* (2nd edn). Columbus: Charles E. Merrill.

Owens, R. (1988). Cognition and language in the mentally retarded population. In M. Beveridge, G. Conti-Ramsden & I. Leudar (eds), *Language and communication in mentally handicapped people*. London: Chapman and Hall.

Owens, R.E. & MacDonald, J.D. (1982). Communicative uses of the early speech of non-delayed and Down syndrome children. *American Journal of Mental Deficiency 86*, 503–11.

Prutting, C.A., Bagshaw, N., Goldstein, H., Juskowitz, S. & Umen, I. (1978). Clinician–child discourse: Some preliminary questions. *Journal of Speech and Hearing Disorders 43*, 115–22.

Prutting, C.A. & Kirchner, D.M. (1983). Applied pragmatics. In T.M. Gallagher & C.A. Prutting (eds), *Pragmatic assessment and intervention issues in language*. San Diego: College Hill Press.

Rice, M.L. & Sell, M.A. (1990). The social interactive coding system: Language, speech and hearing services in schools. *American Speech-language-hearing Association 21*, 2–14.

Rice, M.L., Sell, M.A. & Hadley, P.M. (1988). *Social interactive skills of language impaired preschoolers*. Manuscript in preparation. Lawrence: University of Kansas.

Schiefelbusch, R.L. (1980) (ed.). *Non speech language and communication: Analysis and intervention*. Baltimore: University Park Press.

Smith, D.W. (1982). *Recognisable patterns of human malformation*. Philadelphia: Saunders.

Snow, C. (1977). Mothers' speech research: From input to interaction. In E.E. Snow & C.A. Ferguson (eds), *Talking to children: Language input and acquisition*. London: Cambridge University Press.

Snyder, L. (1975). Pragmatics in language-deficient children: Prelinguistic and early verbal performatives and presuppositions. PhD thesis. University of Colorado.

Stern, D. (1971). A microanalysis of mother–infant interaction. *Journal of the American Academy of Child Psychiatry 10*, 501–17.

Stern, D. (1974). Mother and infant at play: The dyadic interaction involving facial, vocal and gaze behaviours. In M. Lewis & L. Rosenblum (eds), *The effect of the infant on its caregiver*. New York: John Wiley & Sons.

Stern, D., Jaffe, J., Beebe, B. & Bennett, S. (1975). Vocalising in unison and in alternation: Two modes of communication within the mother–infant dyad. In D. Aronson & R. Rieber (eds), Developmental psycholinguistic and communication disorders. *Annals of the New York Academy of Sciences 263*, 89–100.

Tiegerman, E. & Siperstein, M. (1984). Individual patterns of interaction in the mother–child dyad: Implications for the language-disordered child. *Topics in Language Disorders 4*, 50–62.

Wells, G. (1981). Becoming a communicator. In G. Wells (ed.), *Learning through interaction: The study of language development*. Cambridge: Cambridge University Press.

Wood, B.S. (1981). *Children and communication: Verbal and nonverbal language development* (2nd edn). Englewood Cliffs: Prentice-Hall.

Chapter 4

Selection of Initial Vocabularies for Use in Manual Sign Language Programs

Kathleen Dice
West Kempsey Public School
Kempsey, NSW

One of the most perplexing problems facing special educators working with school-aged children who have developmental disability is how to assist them to communicate more effectively. The majority of children with severe and profound developmental disability communicate very little or not at all verbally (Luftig, 1982, p 81). Typically, the speech they do possess is characterised by single-word utterances, purposeless repetitions or unintelligibility. Of the personal, interpersonal and community living skills that are important for this population (see Figure 4-1), communication is one that challenges the confidence and instructional planning capability of most special educators.

The use of augmentative communication systems is now widespread owing to the increased recognition that they provide an effective means of communication for individuals whose speech is inadequate for that purpose. Among augmentative communication systems, manual sign language has been one of the most popular for use with persons who have severe and profound developmental disabilities (Luftig, 1984). Manual sign language has been defined by Poulton and Algozzine (1980) as "communication accomplished by positioning the hands in space relative to the body" (p 146). It includes both signs and commonly understood gestures (Jones, 1980). Instructors of manual sign language always say the word as they model the sign and encourage the learner to do the same. Many advantages of using manual sign language have been reported in the literature. These

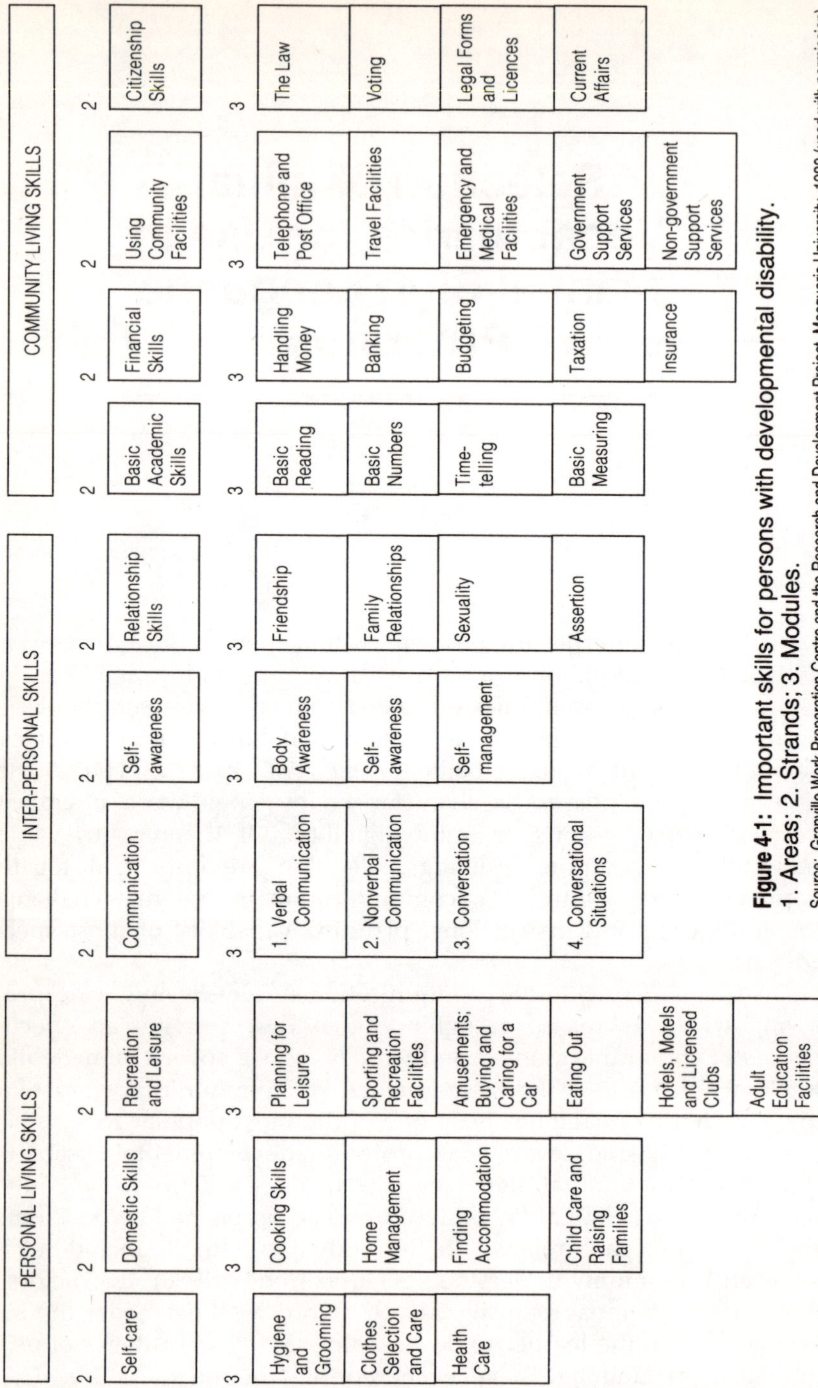

Figure 4-1: Important skills for persons with developmental disability.
1. Areas; 2. Strands; 3. Modules.
Source: Granville Work Preparation Centre and the Research and Development Project, Macquarie University, 1980 (used with permission).

include improved communication, spontaneous use of signs, facilitation of speech development, positive changes in behaviour, improved eye contact, attention, motivation and social interaction.

In Australia and New Zealand the signs taught are taken from the *Dictionary of Australasian Signs* (Jeanes, Reynolds & Coleman, 1989). This source, originally designed for persons with severe hearing impairment, contains more than two thousand signs. Individuals with severe or profound developmental disability are not likely to learn more than a very small number of these because of the limitations of memory and intellect that characterise their disability. These limitations must be taken into consideration when planning initial lexicons for this population. A key aim must be to select a minimum of vocabulary items which will have maximum communicative value for the learner. The importance of these initial items is all the more emphasised by the fact that their communicative value is a critical determiner of the ongoing success of the learner's manual sign communication program (Blau, 1983, p 212; Carlson, 1981, p 240; Reichle, Williams & Ryan, 1981, p 50).

If the purpose of intervention is to achieve effective and efficient communication for the learner, too much is being left to chance by selecting vocabulary items on the basis of intuition. This has all too often been the case (Luftig, 1983, p 279). Rather, informed decision-making on the part of special educators is called for. The best source of information to guide decision-making is the recent empirical literature and its accompanying theory base, for it has been demonstrated that most language and communication intervention efforts that have achieved success have been structured around recent psycholinguistic research and theory (Bryen & Joyce, 1985, p 33). At no time in the past has the literature advocated such a decisive approach toward vocabulary selection. Those special educators who are knowledgeable about current trends are in a better position than ever to obtain optimum results from intervention time invested.

This chapter seeks to present a concise view of current theory on vocabulary selection procedures for special educators and to bring to their attention some of the best practices on offer that comply with that theory. Of course, the point should be made at the outset that signing is not necessarily the most appropriate communication system for all nonverbal children with developmental disability. For some, the cognitive demands involved in representing various meaning classes by spoken or gestural symbolic systems may be just too great. Discussion of non-symbolic alternative communication systems is beyond the scope of this chapter but may be found in Bloomberg and Johnson (1991), Musselwhite and St Louis (1982) and Siegel-Causey and Guess (1989). See also Chapters 7 and 8.

Vocabulary Selection Procedures

When beginning a manual sign communication program with a child who has severe or profound developmental disability, single words/signs are a good place to start. The initial manual sign vocabulary will consist largely of one-sign expressions (considered as utterances) with each sign representing a complete word or concept (Moores, 1974, p 387). Some children will progress to two-sign utterances, whereby they simply link already known words/signs. The one- and two-word stages of communication development (see Stages 3 and 4(1) in Table 4-1) are the ones with which special educators implementing an augmentative communication system like manual sign language are most concerned.

The idea that designing an initial sign lexicon for a learner depends on informed judgement has already been alluded to. Three kinds of knowledge enter into the decision-making process according to Fristoe and Lloyd (1980, p 170):

1. Knowledge of child language acquisition
2. Knowledge of manual signs and linguistic constraints and their use
3. Knowledge of the needs and desires of the individual for whom the lexicon is intended.

All guidelines for vocabulary selection relate back to these three categories of knowledge which the literature more commonly has referred to as developmental, motoric and functional knowledge. The

Table 4-1: Stages in learning to talk.

Preverbal Stage	Uncontrolled vocalising
Stage 1	Meaningful interaction with people and objects Looking together / Turn-taking and imitation / Appropriate play
Stage 2	Preverbal skills: (1) Performatives (2) Protowords
Stage 3	First words
Stage 4	Combining words into sentences: (1) Putting two words together (2) Early sentences
Stage 5	Extending meaning

Source: S. Bochner, P. Price & L. Salamon (1988) (used with permission).

significance of these three knowledge bases with regard to vocabulary selection for manual sign language programs is explained with reference to three generic theoretical principles as follows:

Selecting a Functional Vocabulary for the Learner

Recent empirical literature has recommended that the selection of a functional vocabulary be the goal of communication intervention (Duchan, 1988, p 147; Kaiser, Alpert & Warren, 1987, p 248; Warren & Rogers-Warren, 1985, p 5). It matters little how many words/signs an individual learns to imitate if they cannot be used communicatively. A vocabulary item that is functional for an individual is one that can be used to influence other people. This usually entails some manipulation of the environment, with the partner in the communication exchange (such as mother, teacher or aide) acting as the agent in carrying out the signer's instruction or request, or merely responding socially to the child. If the learner has signs on command that afford even a limited amount of power to control environmental events, then the learning of manual signs will be more successful (Bryen, Goldman & Quinlisk-Gill, 1988, p 135; Johnson, 1986, p 52; Warren & Rogers-Warren, 1985, p 6). This finding is well demonstrated in an example recorded by Kopchick and Lloyd (1976, p 517) who were reporting on the success of a 24-hour total communication program in an institutional setting.

> Within a week, communication had increased dramatically. Some of the clients enjoyed asking staff members for things just to see them active. It was as if they had found a power that they never had before. They learned that it was easier to manipulate people through specific and structured gestures than to scream and pound tables.

Leeming, Swann, Coupe and Mittler (1979, p 263) reported a similar effect after teaching a student just three meaningful and relevant signs.

> On her return to school in the new year after a two-week holiday Susan seemed so desperate to communicate that her speech development was quite remarkable. She used her signs for "drink" and "piano" immediately after she entered the classroom. Within a short time during an individual session she began to repeat words quite distinctly. In fact, she imitated thirty spoken words during this short space of time. Her delight and excitement were immeasurable . . .

Examples abound to support the effectiveness of functionally useful vocabulary items in promoting communication and in extending the learners' active participation in controlling the happenings of their own lives. With functional usefulness being regarded as the most predominant basis for selecting initial vocabulary (Blau, 1983, p 213; Kaiser et al, 1987, p 264; Karlan & Lloyd, 1983, p 15), it goes without saying that every learner needs an individualised initial vocabulary (Johnson, 1986, p 47; Kiernan, Reid & Goldbart, 1987, p 78). Vocabulary items that are functionally useful or appropriate for one learner are not likely to be so for another, so different are the etiologies as well as the life experiences of these children. The need for economy in the number of items composing an initial lexicon suggests that the inclusion of any item must be justified according to its value in assisting the learner to communicate what he or she wants to say. To include items that the learner does not need is likely to be time-consuming and non-productive in terms of promoting the learner's communicative behaviour (Kiernan et al, 1987, p 78).

Considering Developmental Data when Planning an Initial Lexicon

Much of the knowledge base that has accumulated on language and communication development in normal children can be applied with good effect to children with developmental disability. Previous controversy surrounding this issue has now given way to greater acceptance of the premise that children with developmental disability or delay acquire language in the same general manner and sequence as normal children do, although at a much reduced rate (Bochner, Price & Salamon, 1988, p 1; McLean & Snyder-McLean, 1987, p 92). Developmental data provide a useful guide for decision-making about the kinds of language structures or expressive meanings that it would be usual for a child of comparable development to be learning and capable of attaining (Blau, 1983, p 209; Winitz, 1983, p 33). Such data can perhaps best be viewed as being complementary to a knowledge of the learner's functional vocabulary needs. Lucas' (1980, p 1) summary is representative of the widely held theoretical view that:

> . . . the remediation process for language disorders should be approached from what is known about normal development, with the knowledge from normal development being blended with what is known about each exceptional child's special needs.

Special educators are well advised to use developmental data as a guide, but they must take responsibility for determining what language is taught and when, largely on the basis of each learner's particular learning characteristics and functional requirements (McCormick & Goldman, 1984, p 211; Musselwhite & St Louis, 1982, p 26; Reichle & Keogh, 1985, p 27).

Considering System Constraints on Vocabulary Selection and Teaching Order

No augmentative communication system offers the convenience of spoken language. Each system's unique features will in some way constrain the ease of learning particular vocabulary items. Manual sign language's unique constraining features include its requirements of physical production and visual comprehension of signs. Some signs will be easier to produce and/or comprehend than others, and this should be a consideration when planning the order of introducing signs, selected for their functional usefulness, into the communication program (Karlan & Lloyd, 1983, p 21). Naturally, teaching easy-to-produce and/or easy-to-comprehend signs initially should facilitate sign acquisition and greatly increase the likelihood of the learner acquiring an effective means of communication (Kohl, 1981, p 402).

The significance of the three knowledge bases for vocabulary selection has been explained. These knowledge bases can now be examined in greater detail, the objective being to highlight, for each, those empirical guidelines that contribute toward informed decision-making at the one- and two-word utterance stages.

Section 1: Knowledge of Child Language Acquisition

The importance of function in child language acquisition cannot be emphasised enough. Children learn words, according to Bloom (1973), because they code regularly recurring experiences in their lives and because words enable them to communicate their needs and wants to others. Indeed, the words that children utter always have some function (Rees, 1978, p 516), so that function is perhaps the most important factor in lexicon planning. Documentation of the functions of children's language began with Bloom's (1973) observation that all the words children use at the single-word utterance stage are of two functional types: substantive and relational. Substantive words are words that name objects (such as Mummy) or classes of objects (such as dog) (Wood, 1981, p 91). Names of persons are the most frequently used of the substantive words, particularly "Mum", "Dad" and the child's name, or variations of these (Bloom, 1973, p 92; Leeming et al, 1979, p 119). Substantive words can have various functions (such as agent, object or possession) (Woolman, 1974, p 329).

Relational words comprise a smaller proportion of words in the young child's vocabulary, but they are used individually with far greater frequency than words of the substantive type (Wood, 1981, p 91). Relational words refer to relationships between objects. Included are verbs ("cry"), adjectives ("big") and prepositions ("away") (Lahey & Bloom, 1977, p 342). The major relational words at the single-word stage and the functions they code have been listed by Bloom (1973) (see Table 4-2).

Planning a Lexicon

When planning an initial one-word lexicon, provision must be made for the inclusion of substantive and relational words. In the functional, individualised programs that are currently being advocated, substantive words are selected with sensitivity to individual differences and varieties of situation (Bloom, 1970, p 227; Byler, 1985, p 112; Moerk, 1977, p 124). Procedures for selecting substantive words will be explained in detail in Section 2 which deals with functional aspects of vocabulary selection. As for relational words, one word to code each of the listed relational functions in Table 4-2 might be included in the initial lexicon as these are highly useful, heavy-duty words for any learner. (Note that some words code more than one function and only need to be listed once.) Other less important relational words which are functional for the individual concerned can be selected in the same way that substantive words are selected.

Some recommendations for the inclusion or exclusion of particular substantive or relational words or word groups have appeared in the literature and are important for the lexicon planner. This information is now summarised.

At the one-word utterance stage, the ideas encoded in personal pronouns can be represented through the use of nominal forms (person, object and place names) (Fristoe & Lloyd, 1980, p 173). This

Table 4-2: Major relational words and their apparent meanings as one-word utterances.

General relationship	Word	Function/meaning
Existence	there	To point out objects
	uh-oh	To point out objects — particularly those that startled the child
Recurrence	more	First to request and later to comment on the recurrence of an activity or object
Disappearance	away	To comment on the disappearance of object that had existed in context
	A' gone	(Same as above)
Non-existence	no 1	To comment on non-existence where existence had been expected
Cessation	stop	To comment on the cessation of an activity
Rejection	no 2	To protest undesired action or comment on forbidden object (such as stove)
Action	up 1	To request the action of being picked up
Location	up 2	To comment on spatial location

Source: L. Bloom (1973) (used with permission).

seems preferable because personal pronouns rarely occur in children's vocabularies at this stage, and the shifting speaker/hearer distinction is a difficult one to teach (Lahey & Bloom, 1977, p 344).

At the two-word utterance stage, young children either continue to use nominal forms (such as "Peter push") or transfer to using predominantly pronominal forms (such as "Me push") (Lahey & Bloom, p 344). The developmental data suggest that, although personal pronouns might be introduced at the two-word utterance stage, programming should remain flexible to accommodate these individual preferences (Byler, 1985, p 113).

Other Semantic Categories

Forms that code the manifestations of *internal states* (such as "cry", "hug" and "eat") are more easily taught and learned than forms that code the states themselves (such as "sad", "love" and "hungry"). This is because learners have difficulty making form/content inductions about concepts that are not externally tangible (Lahey & Bloom, p 344). Words that code internal states can be introduced at the two-word stage when the child is beginning to combine words to express relationships.

Colour attribution is not typically found in children's early language productions until the emergence of multiple-word utterances (Lahey & Bloom, p 347). Neither do colour words have much communicative value. Colour is rarely mentioned by persons except to contrast two identical objects, and the use of colour words is too limited to justify their inclusion at this level (Fristoe & Lloyd, 1980, p 174). Colours do not have the broad topical reference that some other adjectives have (such as "big" and "hot") (Karlan & Lloyd, 1983, p 15). Blau (1983, p 227) has suggested that an exception might be made in specific cases, for example, if a learner's identification of an item by colour combined with eye pointing can significantly improve his communication.

Polar opposites are pairs of antonyms (primarily modifiers such as "hot"/"cold", "big"/"little" and "happy"/"sad") reflecting contrasts of related concepts (Blau, p 226). Data from normal language development suggest that children tend to learn the more salient attribute, or marked member, of a pair of polar opposites first (such as "big", "heavy", "hot" and "dirty"), and they refer to the unmarked member by use of "no" + attribute (such as "no big") (Lahey & Bloom, 1977, p 347). To avoid confusing the learner by introducing two words (such as "hot"/"cold") for what may be one concept of heat, the unmarked member might be excluded from instruction initially (Karlan & Lloyd, 1983, p 15). For older children, however, some flexibility is advised, particularly if the learner has frequent need for each item in the pair or has difficulty combining items like "not big". For this group, Fristoe and Lloyd (1980, quoted in Blau, 1983, p 226) have recommended inclusion generally for pairs of items frequently used or directly related to basic bodily needs.

There is consensus that "*no*" is an extremely useful item functionally in an initial lexicon. Other than being a response to a direct question, and this is not a function for "no" normally used in signing contexts (Fristoe & Lloyd, 1980, p 174), "no" serves a variety of communicative functions (such as rejection, denial and non-existence) that are important to young children (Lahey & Bloom, 1977, p 345). "No" also offers many possibilities for combination with substantive and relational words at the two-word utterance stage (Blau, p 227; Karlan & Lloyd, p 15).

Lahey and Bloom (p 345) argued that "*yes*" should be excluded from initial lexicons on the grounds that in normal children's language development it functions communicatively only as a response to a question or to signal agreement with the statement of another. As most utterances are statements that affirm something (such as "telephone" and "sore"), it is unnecessary to say "yes" unless the truth of a statement is questioned (for example, "Is it sore?" "Yes.") Yet several writers have recommended the building of an appropriate "yes"/"no" response early in training to provide the learner with an immediate means of environmental control (Alberto, Garrett, Briggs & Unberger, 1983, p 10; Byler, 1985, p 113; Keogh & Reichle, 1985, p 187; Silverman, 1980, p 81). It would seem that the special educator is left to grapple with the decision as to whether to include "yes" for a particular learner. It does seem advisable, though, to teach "no" first, because of its functional usefulness and to prevent any confusion that might result from teaching "no" and "yes" together. For adolescent learners, the inclusion of "yes" has been considered appropriate.

It has been recommended that "want" be the first *action word* taught (Reichle & Keogh, 1985, p 28). "Want" is a key word for expressing desires, and the expression of desires appears to be one of the earliest linguistic functions mastered by both normal infants and non-speaking children (Schaeffer, 1980a, p 56). Schaeffer (p 40) has related that learners appear to express desires in signs sooner and more easily than they learn to describe or to ask questions, and they appear to prefer to express desires rather than to describe or ask. The early inclusion of "want" also gives the learner a means of differentiating between object identification and object requests (that is, "apple" is differentiated from "want apple") (Keogh & Reichle, 1982, quoted in Alberto et al, 1983, p 10).

After "want", "go" is suggested as the second most important *action word*. It is the most frequent mover-location action verb produced by children during the initial stages of language acquisition (Bloom, Miller & Hood, 1978, quoted in Alberto et al, 1983, p 10).

Fristoe and Lloyd (1980, p 174) suggested that *wh-question words* be postponed until the two-word utterance stage. Their reasoning was that, although some children do use wh-question words, notably "what" and "where", at the one-word stage in spoken language (Nelson, 1973), these functions could be achieved just as efficiently through the use of facial expression, gesture and/or direction of gaze, so that these words need not be introduced until later.

Organisation of the Lexicon

Hypothetically, knowledge of the developmental and functional information presented so far, along with knowledge of the functional information contained in Part Two of this chapter, would have enabled the special educator to accumulate an initial pool of substantive and relational words customised to suit the learner's functional requirements. What would then appear to be needed would be some way to organise these words into a convenient instructional framework. Lahey and Bloom (1977) have provided such a framework. Their organisation of a first lexicon, structured with regard to language content (that is, substantive and relational words and the functions they code), has served as a model for subsequent lexical advances (for example, Fristoe & Lloyd, 1980; Karlan & Lloyd, 1983) (see Table 4-3).

In the left-hand column of Lahey and Bloom's model lexicon are the content categories which are represented by single-word utterances (Bloom, 1970, 1973). Provision has been made in subsequent columns for relational words. These have been divided into two groups according to their specificity, a feature that can be used to good advantage when selecting initial language targets. Those major relational words that can be used to refer to many different objects (such as "no" and "more") are recorded in column two. Of the relational words, these have the most potential for communication in many different situations. Those relational words that are more specific to objects but still relate to many objects are recorded in column three. Some of these words are more specific to objects than others. For example, Lahey and Bloom (1977) have explained that "give", "get", "make" and "fall" can refer to more objects than "eat" and "throw". "Big" and "dirty" (included) can refer to more objects than "orange" and "round" (excluded). Like the substantive words to be recorded in column four, relational words that are more specific to objects are chosen to reflect learner interests or the frequency with which the learner comes into contact with particular people, objects, actions and so on. Clearly, the Lahey and Bloom lexicon model offers a great deal

Table 4-3: Organisation of a first lexicon by content and form.

Content category	Form		
	Relational words		Substantive words
	Relational words that are not object specific	Relational words that are more specific to objects but still relate to many objects	
Rejection	no		
Non-existence or disappearance	no, all gone, away		
Cessation of action	stop, no		
Prohibition of action	no		
Recurrence of objects, actions on objects	more, again, another		
Noting existent of or identifying objects	this, there, that		
Actions on objects		give, do, make, get, throw, eat, wash, kiss	
Actions involved in locating objects/self		put, up, down sit, fall, go	
Attributes or descriptions of objects		big, hot, dirty, heavy	
Persons associated with objects (as in possession); names			person

Source: Lahey & Bloom (1977) (used with permission).

of flexibility in its approach to individualising vocabulary selection at the one-word stage.

This flexibility continues as the learner progresses to the two-word stage. At the two-word stage, the content categories that code the language functions are the same; they are common to all child language (Bloom, 1970; Brown, 1973; Schlesinger, 1971). Now however, the learner uses two words instead of one to express each function. The two-word combinations are formed by using a variety of combinations of the previously learned substantive and relational functions (Woolman, 1974, p 330). Table 4-4 illustrates the two-word combinations (see "Form") that code the language functions, and gives an example of each.

While the Lahey and Bloom lexicon model (Table 4-3) serves mainly as an organisational structure for single words, categorising them according to their content and form, it makes no provision for listing the two-word combinations to be taught initially. It is suggested,

Table 4-4: Semantic relations expressed in early two-word combinations.

Semantic relation	Form	Possible context	Example
Existence	relational word + object name (introducer + entity)	Child calls attention to an object or picture of an object by pointing	"this car" "it ball"
Negation (three meanings): non-existence, rejection or denial	relational word + object name (negation + entity)	If indicating *non-existence*, child may be searching for a lost cookie; if *rejection*, child may be refusing an offer of a cookie; if *denial*, child may be responding to the question "Is this your cookie?"	"no cookie"
Recurrence	relational word + object name (more + entity)	Child indicates awareness of the reappearance of an object or the desire for an additional amount (or a new instance) of something.	"more juice" "more swing"
Attribution	adjective + noun (attribute + entity)	Child calls attention to some characteristic of an object.	"big ball" "pretty baby"
Possession	noun + noun, or pronoun + noun	Child indicates (by pointing to or holding up) someone's property.	"Mummy sock" "my coat"
Locative (two types): action or entity	verb + noun/pronoun (action + locative), noun/pronoun + verb (locative + action), or noun + noun (entity + locative)	Child indicates a movement occurring in a specific place or child indicates that an object exists in a particular place.	"sit beach" or "sweater chair"
Agent-action	noun/pronoun + verb	Child indicates the initiator of an action and the movement.	"mummy go" "doggie run"
Action-object	verb + noun/pronoun	Child indicates a movement or process with someone or something receiving it.	"hit ball" "drink juice"
Agent-object	noun/pronoun + noun/pronoun	Child indicates someone or something in direct interaction with another person or thing.	"daddy ball" "Mummy baby"

Source: McCormick (1990) (used with permission).

therefore, that a separate format for listing the two-word combinations would be complementary to the one-word lexicon. The heading "Example" in Table 4-4 might easily be changed to "Two-word combinations to be taught" to provide such a format. Any number of two-word combinations could then be listed for each content category, with words from the one-word lexicon coding the required language functions. A number of special educators (such as Bochner et al, 1988; Cole & Cole, 1981; Lombardino et al, 1981; Stremel-Campbell et al, 1977) have listed two-word combinations intended for instruction by referring to the developmentally based content categories for two-word combinations. However, no consistent format has been used. Taken together, the Lahey and Bloom lexicon model and a format for listing two-word combinations according to their language functions provide an effective approach to vocabulary selection. This approach adheres to developmental recommendations for language content and is at the same time highly functional and individualised. Such a model fits in well with current theoretical leanings.

Some Sample Lexicons

Having presented structural frameworks for organising the one-word and two-word functions that have been selected for the learner, it might now prove helpful to examine some of the examples of core lexicons that have been proposed. This is not to suggest that the words contained in any particular lexicon are to be adopted generally as being suitable for all handicapped learners. Rather, it is to acknowledge that careful consideration has gone into word choices in the past and that building on the expertise of others who have gone before seems a somewhat more sensible approach than starting from scratch. Sample lexicons might serve as references for special educators planning individualised lexicons. Does the lexicon, for example, seem to contain a reasonable number of words? Do the words seem to be of the appropriate sort? At this stage of the lexicon planning, some of the word frequency data (collected by, for example, Gillham, 1979; Walker, 1984) may be referred to; it is not suggested that items be deliberately selected from that resource pool but, rather, that the data serve as a cross-check on the value of including those items that have already been selected on the basis of their functional usefulness for the learner.

Holland (1975) was perhaps the first to attempt to devise a sample core lexicon. It consisted of words that were common to early child language as well as items that were functionally useful for the learner. Holland presented a rationale for the inclusion of each word in her sample lexicon so that other special educators could judge the merits of her selections in accordance with their learners' requirements.

Lahey and Bloom (1977) reviewed Holland's suggestions. They disagreed with some and made recommendations for the exclusion of these in the light of their knowledge of the developmental data. Their recommendations along with those of other researchers in the field are contained above in Table 4-3. Refinement of Holland's lexicon in accordance with Lahey and Bloom's recommendations would suggest that the following items are potentially useful in an initial lexicon:

- the child's own name
- the names of significant others
- a concrete action indicating a basic desire, like "hug"
- "want"
- "wash"
- "more"
- "go"
- "no"
- a favourite food
- a word used to express a negative emotion or dislike, like "yuck"
- "gone"
- a loved activity
- "up"
- "down", being among the most frequent relational words
- "there"
- "that"
- "hi"
- "big" or other attribute choices
- the names of objects important to the individual.

The next advance in lexicon planning came as a response to the realisation that normal development had served as the source of words for both the Holland and the Lahey and Bloom lexicons. Those writers had formulated their lexicons for children who were language-delayed. Although it is now known that the developmental data are equally applicable to both populations, Fristoe and Lloyd (1980) reasoned that a lexicon based on frequency of word use by people with developmental delay would be more appropriate for them. As part of their strategy, Fristoe and Lloyd (1979) had earlier selected the 50 words/signs that occurred most frequently in 20 sign language manuals used for people with developmental delay. It was their belief that the high frequency of the occurrence of these words in sign manuals could be interpreted to mean that they were especially useful for persons with developmental delay, or were easy to teach. On the basis of Holland's (1975) rationales and the recommendations of Lahey and Bloom (Table 4-4), Fristoe and Lloyd (1980) then added and deleted signs to arrive at the sample lexicon in Table 4-5.

Just how appropriate Fristoe and Lloyd's sample core lexicon would

Table 4-5: Fristoe and Lloyd's sample core lexicon for persons with developmental delay.

Content category	Form		
	Relational signs		Substantive signs
	Signs that are not object specific	Signs relating to many objects	
Rejection	negative		
Non-existence or disappearance	negative, all gone		
Cessation of action	negative, stop		
Prohibition of action	negative		
Recurrence of objects and actions on objects	more		
Noting existence of or identifying objects	this/that/those		
Actions on objects		bring, drink, eat, get, give, make, open, play, throw, wash	
Actions involved in locating objects or self		fall, go, put, sit, stand, run, walk, up, down	
Attributes or descriptions of objects		bad, big, broken, dirty, good, happy, heavy, hot, open	
Persons and animals associated with objects (as in possession)			baby, big, bird, cat, dog, father, girl, hat, mother, you and name signs
Other objects named			Apple, ball, bathroom/toilet/potty, book, candy, car, chair/sit, coat, comb, cookie, cup, door, drink, eat/food, house, milk, pants, school, shirt, shoe(s), sock, spoon, TV, table, water

Source: Fristoe & Lloyd (1980) (used with permission).

be for persons with developmental disability remained to be seen. There was some concern that a lexicon based on secondary data (that is, the frequency of a word's occurrence in sign manuals) rather than on systematic information collection might not be communicatively useful for persons with severe or profound developmental disability in their natural environments. Karlan and Lloyd (1983) therefore set out to investigate the appropriateness of the lexicon with regard to both children and adolescents/adults. The social validation study that they conducted involved subjective evaluation of each lexicon item. Fifty-seven teachers and speech therapists judged the appropriateness of the lexicon items for *elementary-aged,* severely handicapped children they worked with. Forty-three parents, teachers, teaching assistants, speech therapists, vocational trainers, group-home trainers and staff, and institutional direct-care staff judged the appropriateness of the lexicon items for the severely handicapped *adolescents and adults* they worked with. Each respondent indicated whether the item was judged to be essential to, useful in, could be useful in or of no value in an initial expressive vocabulary.

The results of the social validation study gave substantial support to the initial core lexicon sample produced by Fristoe and Lloyd for use with both the elementary and adolescent/adult groups generally (Karlan & Lloyd, p 18). None of the items was considered to be of no value, and few were placed in the questionable, or could be useful, category. It would appear that the Fristoe and Lloyd sample core lexicon (see Table 4-6) has some validity as an indicator of words that might be included in initial lexicons for children (including adolescents) with developmental delay. Cooney's (1985, p 17) observation that the Fristoe and Lloyd lexicon shares many items (approximately 100 words) with the first three stages of the Makaton Vocabulary, a lexicon first developed in England and revised in Australia to meet the particular communication needs of people with intellectual disability (Walker, 1984), would seem to support that view. Further, Karlan and Lloyd felt that the subdivision of the Fristoe and Lloyd lexicon into *essential* and *useful* vocabulary items (see Tables 4-6 and 4-7) could prove to be helpful when planning intervention, especially when establishing important early communication priorities.

As indicated above, Karlan and Lloyd investigated the particular age-appropriateness of Fristoe and Lloyd's lexicon. They had observed

Table 4-6: The Fristoe and Lloyd sample core lexicon: Items within the essential vocabulary range.

Source	*Items*
Elementary survey sample	Dad, Mummy
Adolescent survey sample	angry/mad, clean, cold, come, in, open, sad, shirt, shoes, walk, wash, work, you
Both	bathroom/toilet/potty, bed/sleep, coat, drink, eat/food, go, good, happy, help, hot, look/watch, milk, more, name, no, sign, stop, water

Source: Karlan & Lloyd (1983) (used with permission).

Table 4-7: The Fristoe and Lloyd sample core lexicon: Items within the useful vocabulary range.

Source	*Items*
Elementary survey sample	clean, cold, come, door, in, open, sad, shirt, shoes, wash, you
Adolescent survey sample	Daddy/Father, do, have, heavy, man, money, Mummy/Mother, pat, possess, this/that/those, woman
Both	afraid, all gone/used up/finished, angry/mad, bad, ball, book, boy, break/broken, candy, car, chair/sit, comb, cookie, cry, cup, dirty, down, fall, get, girl, give, hat, house, make, now, on, pants, play, run, school, sock, spoon, stand, table, TV, throw, under, up, what, who

Source: Karlan & Lloyd (1983) (used with permission).

that many of the items in the Fristoe and Lloyd lexicon appeared on face value to be more appropriate for younger severely handicapped learners than for older ones. They set themselves the goal of designing a sample core lexicon that would be more appropriate for adolescent/adult learners. To accomplish this task, they conducted a further systematic survey in which they interviewed the 43 original survey respondents for the adolescent/adult lexicon items. These respondents, prior to exposure to the Fristoe and Lloyd lexicon and rating scale, were asked to provide all the words that would be important for an initial expressive vocabulary. To assist them with the selections, the following content categories were suggested: persons, places, objects, relations (such as "no", "more", "bye"), actions, emotions, food, play/recreation/toys, personal hygiene, vocational, independent living/mobility, other. Fifty-two of Fristoe and Lloyd's 83 items were suggested by more than 25% of the Karlan and Lloyd (1983) respondents. This indicated a substantial overlap with the Fristoe and Lloyd lexicon (Table 4-5), further substantiating the validity of using some of the items from that source with adolescents who were developmentally delayed. However, some differences were also highlighted. Firstly, Karlan and Lloyd's survey had yielded items additional to the Fristoe and Lloyd lexicon, which were noticeably adolescent-oriented. For example, the importance of personal hygiene and vocational or recreational activities was reflected in the inclusion of the items soap, shampoo, toothbrush, toothpaste, deodorant, money, coffee, hamburger, workshop/work area, break/breaktime, restaurant and bowling. Other items (such as "clean", "cold", "work"), which would ordinarily be excluded from an initial lexicon on the grounds of their being developmentally inappropriate, had been nominated. The social validation study had already verified this latter finding. In it, "where", "what" and "money" as well as the above three items had been judged functionally useful for adolescents. (These words had been included for validation in addition to the items from the Fristoe and Lloyd lexicon.)

Clearly, adolescents have functional needs that override the developmental guidelines suitable for younger learners. Karlan and Lloyd (1983, p 18) commented on this point:

> These findings indicate that while various items might not be developmentally appropriate for the initial lexicon, perceived functional need must also be considered. With chronologically older individuals, it may be appropriate to include unmarked opposites such as "clean" or "cold" or developmentally infrequent items such as "work" or "money". The longer experiential history of the persons or the functional frequency of the item might mitigate the problems present with developmentally and chronologically young individuals.

Thus, discretion must always be exercised when deciding how best to balance developmental and functional considerations for older learners. Clearly, Karlan and Lloyd succeeded in showing that a lexicon designed for adolescents would be different from one designed for younger children.

The sample core lexicons that have been discussed here have served to illustrate the organisational structure of first lexicons and to stimulate thinking about the kind of content they should have. In reviewing the approaches of the major contributors to research on lexicon development, it has become evident that, while there is some agreement about specific words that might be useful in an initial lexicon (particularly about relational words that are not object-specific, like "no" and "more"; about high frequency relational words that are more specific, like "big" and "dirty"; and about high frequency substantive words like "Mum" and "drink"), generally lexicons must remain flexible enough to accommodate the needs and interests of individual learners if they are to meet communication needs effectively. The discussion will now turn to those more functional aspects of vocabulary selection that relate to determining what the learner's needs and interests are.

Section 2: Knowledge of the Needs and Interests of the Individual for Whom the Lexicon is Intended

An ecological inventory approach toward vocabulary selection has been recommended as the most efficient and effective way to promote communication and to lead the learner toward independence (Leeming et al, 1979, p 159; McCormick & Schiefelbusch, 1990, p 111). Such an approach entails being knowledgeable about: (1) strategies for determining lexicon items that are functional for learners; and (2) procedures for facilitating systematic data collection of functional lexicon items, referred to as the ecological inventory. By applying functional strategies while at the same time adhering to procedures for observing and recording the learner's interactive behaviour with his or her environment, a fairly valid diagnostic assessment of the learner's needs and interests is possible.

The functional strategies discussed here are ones that have figured prominently in the literature. While they have not been extensively researched, they have been regarded as the best practices by various special educators writing in the field (Nietupski & Hamre-Nietupski, 1977, p 83). These strategies are reviewed in Figure 4-2.

Familiarity of the Referents

In normal language development, children begin to use language expressively to talk about what they know, and this knowledge is related to their sensorimotor experiences (Nelson, quoted in Bernstein and Tiegerman, 1989, p 13). The same principle applies to children with developmental delay (Kiernan et al, 1987, p 9; McCormick & Schiefelbusch, 1990, p 18; McDonald, 1982, p 120). A child can only be expected to learn labels for actions able to be, performed or for

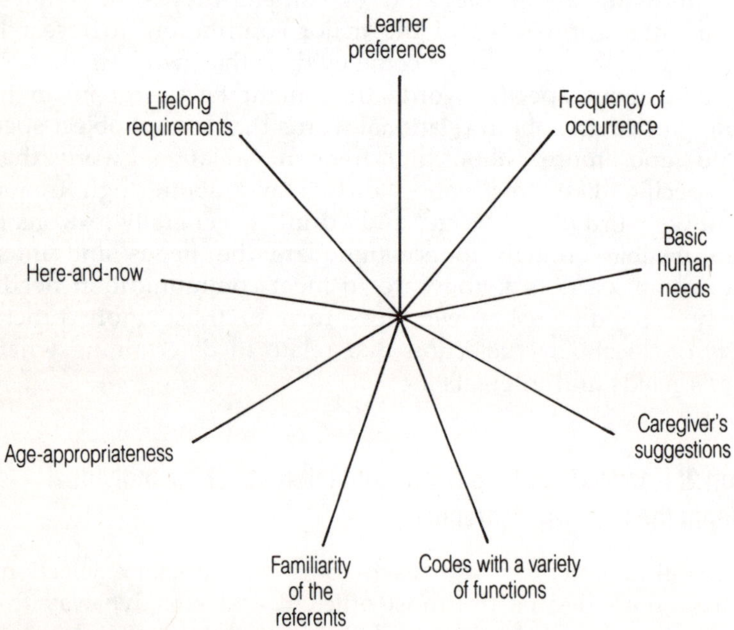

Figure 4-2: Strategies for selecting items that are functional for learners.
Source: Adapted from Hamre-Nietupski et al, 1977.

objects for which mental concepts have been developed (Leeming et al, 1979, p 122), and it is easier to learn signs for these labels (Clarke, Remington & Light, 1986, p 237). The outcome of teaching signs for which the learner has no underlying concept development is likely to be meaningless rote or stimulus-response learning that fails to generalise to communicative use (Leeming et al, 1979, p 103; McLean & Snyder-McLean, 1978, p 13; Romski et al, 1984, p 76).

The way to select referents (that is, the thing that the sign represents) that are familiar to the learner is to observe his or her sensorimotor experiences. The learner's existing repertoire of communicative behaviours (pointing, looking, showing, giving, requesting and so on) should reveal a rich source of potential initial lexicon items (Kaiser et al, 1987, p 260; McDonald, p 91; Russell, 1984, p 66). McLean and Snyder-McLean (1978) have expressed the view that if special educators can be sensitive to learners' conceptions of reality and their crude attempts at communication, they should finally be able to identify vocabulary items which are "real to them, useful to them, and highly possible for them to attain efficaciously and productively" (p 192).

Frequency of Occurrence

A sign for which there is frequent need in the learner's daily life is a sign that will be communicatively useful. Ample opportunities for practice will also enable the sign to be learned more quickly (Cooney, 1985, p 17; Karlan & Lloyd, 1983, p 14), thus contributing to important early success for the learner in the use of an initial signing program. This strategy has received wide support (Warren & Rogers-Warren, 1985, p 9).

Learner Preferences

A particularly powerful strategy is to identify the learner's likes and interests (Hamre-Nietupski et al, 1977, p 106). It is likely that far less effort will need to be expended in the teaching and learning of signs that are motivational for the learner (Reichle et al, 1981, p 53). McLean and Snyder-McLean (1978, p 189) have stated their view that, in the selection of vocabulary items, failure to take sufficient notice of learners' motivations ". . . seems at the least, ill-advised and extremely costly to the overall process of teaching and learning".

Basic Human Needs

Inclusion in the lexicon of vocabulary items related to bodily necessities (such as eating, going to the toilet, bathing and dressing) enables the learner to alert others of personal needs in ways that are socially appropriate. Alberto et al (1983, p 9) have noted that if a child does not have a way to communicate needs, inappropriate behaviours will often result. The occurrence of such behaviours is a clear signal that signs are needed.

Apart from items basic to survival, special educators are becoming aware of the need to include items that will enable the learner to express emotions (such as "yuck!" or "yeh!") (Kiernan et al, 1987, p 76; Porter, 1987, p 93), to engage in social conversation (such as "hi!" and "bye!") (Blau, 1983, pp 221–28) and to execute tasks of daily living (such as shopping and monetary terms) (Meyers et al, 1984, p 65). The basic needs strategy has been one of the most frequently used in traditional intervention programs (Blau, 1983, p 216).

Here-and-now

Selecting vocabulary items from the context of the situations and activities in which the learner is now engaged rather than from the context of the past or future has been regarded as a valuable early strategy (Dayan et al, 1977, p 68; Kiernan et al, 1987, p 76). The developmental data outlined by Wells (1981, p 80) explain the rationale for such an approach.

> Early words tend to refer to the familiar objects in the here-and-now of the child's experience, particularly people, animals, and things that move or cause other things to move, the objects that the child most frequently acts upon, and the actions and states that result from his actions.

Holland, referring to Ashton-Warner's (1971) concept of organicity, which refers to the essential interrelatedness of the child, the word and the activity, stressed the immediacy of children's communicative attempts. In practical terms, this means that vocabulary items selected with regard to the learner's day-to-day active experiences are likely to promote the most effective learning (Bottorf & DePape, 1982, p 64). Routine daily events are an excellent source of vocabulary items.

Codes a Variety of Functions

Items that can serve multiple functions for the learner (such as the relational words, and substantive words like "Mum" which is frequently used to make requests) contribute to the efficiency of an initial lexicon. Included in this strategy would be items that can be used across a variety of settings (Scheuerman et al, 1976) or that can be combined with other items to form two-word combinations (Karlan & Lloyd, 1983, p 15). There has been ample support for this strategy from, for example, Blau, 1983, p 222; Bryen & Joyce, 1985, p 18; Reichle & Keogh, 1985, p 32).

Caregivers' Suggestions

Suggestions of caregivers, based on their knowledge of the child in environments other than the school, can provide a more complete picture of the learner's communication needs. Consideration of caregivers' suggestions should lead to better choices of initial items as well as greater home support for the instructional goals. Additionally, as communication is an interactive process, the needs of the caregiver to transmit information to, or to request choices of, the learner should also to be represented in an initial vocabulary (Blau, 1983, p 214; Kiernan, 1984, p 252). Dennis et al (1982, p 26) have advised that inclusion of caregivers' suggestions be based on their functional utility for both the learner and the caregiver. Professional judgement will ensure that a proper balance is maintained between vocabulary items that the caregiver wants to have the learner communicate and those items that emerge naturally from the learner's activities and interests (Carlson, 1981, p 24).

Lifelong Requirements

Brown, Nietupski and Hamre-Nietupski (1976) were among the first to apply Wolfensberger's (1972) principle of normalisation to communication planning for children with developmental delay. That principle stated that persons with severe handicaps should be prepared for normal existence in mainstream society. In the view of Brown et al (quoted in McCormick & Goldman, 1984, p 211), appropriate vocabulary items to teach learners would be those that maximise their potential for productive and independent functioning in home, community and vocational settings. Consideration of the demands that environments beyond the school are likely to make on the learner will assist special educators' efforts to prioritise those items that will increase the probability of transition to and maintenance in those environments (Bernstein & Tiegerman, 1989, p 195; McCormick & Goldman, 1984, p 218; Reichle & Karlan, 1985, p 52).

Age-appropriateness

When considering how best to prepare a learner to function independently with regard to communication, age should be taken into account. Younger children need to be prepared to function socially with non-handicapped peers in school, home and community environments. Academically, they have the luxury of many years ahead for instruction, so that broad language goals that will enable them to express and understand many different ideas are appropriate (Bowerman, 1978, p 211). An important consideration for younger learners is whether the vocabulary items will help them to be viewed more favourably by others (McCormick & Goldman, p 218).

For older learners whose time in school is limited, there is a greater sense of urgency to narrow programming goals toward the communication requirements of future work, community, recreational and domestic environments (Bernstein & Tiegerman, 1989, p 211; McCormick & Goldman, p 218).

These, then, are the strategies that can be used to select lexicon items that are functional for learners. A single strategy might sometimes be sufficient to recommend the inclusion of an item. If, for example, the item represented an extremely powerful reinforcer, that might be enough to warrant its inclusion (Reichle, Williams & Ryan, 1981, p 54). However, for the selection of a whole list of items, the use of a number of the strategies in combination is recommended (Musselwhite & St Louis, 1982, p 27; Nietupski & Hamre-Nietupski, 1977, p 83; Stremel-Campbell, Cantrell & Halle, 1977, p 340).

Ecological Inventories

The strategies would normally be used in conjunction with an ecological inventory. The purpose of all ecological inventories is the same. They are conducted to determine what it is that the child is trying to communicate by his or her behaviours, or what language could be potentially useful for the learner in the present and projected future environments. A fuller discussion of this approach may be found in Chapter 8 of this volume. Communicated information in the form of sounds or gestures gathered during the ecological inventory is translated into developmentally appropriate words to be used in lexicon planning for the learner. This is best viewed as an ongoing process (Russell, 1984, p 68; Yoder & Kraat, 1983, p 33). Words can be added to and deleted from the learner's lexicon in accordance with changing needs and interests (Montgomery, 1986, p 33). The lexicon remains flexible but, ideally, continues to contain a small number of dynamically useful items as opposed to a large static vocabulary pool (Blau, 1983, p 221; Byler, 1985, p 112; Musselwhite & St Louis, 1982, p 26).

Instructional procedures for conducting ecological inventories and formats for recording the functional data collected have appeared in the literature. For younger children, special educators will find Bochner et al (1988, pp 32–3), Carlson (1981, pp 240–45) and Leeming et al (1979, pp 238–67 and 372–79) particularly helpful for the instructions they provide on how to conduct ecological inventories for non-speaking children, in addition to the discussion in Chapter 8 of the present volume. For older learners, the top-down curriculum strategy described comprehensively by McCormick and Goldman (1984, pp 218–21) and briefly by Miller and Allaire (1987, p 289) is very suitable. As these approaches cannot be adequately described within the limited space of this chapter, special educators may wish to consult the sources themselves for complete coverage of the procedures involved.

Once the initial vocabulary items to be used in communication training have been determined, function will often be the best indicator of when to teach an item. Items are taught as they are needed in naturally occurring situations. This is the approach promoted by current theory (Miller & Allaire, 1987, p 290), with one exception. This is that language function, although an important variable when deciding what to teach and when to teach it, is not the only variable to be considered when communication systems other than speech are being used (Luftig, 1983, p 279; 1984, p 193). When manual sign language is the augmentative system used, motoric factors must be considered as well. The next section examines the motoric aspects of manual sign language communication to see what part they play in the vocabulary selection process.

Section 3: Knowledge of Manual Signs and Constraints on Their Use

In the introduction to this chapter it was pointed out that the ease of learning of manual signs is affected by constraints acting on the system, namely, those of physical production and visual comprehension of signs. Other system constraints considered by Luftig (1984, p 193) include characteristics relating to the referents that the signs represent and those relating to the perceived relationships between the signs and their referents. The following discussion summarises research relating to those considerations.

Physical Production of Signs

1. Formational Characteristics of Signs

Seven bi-polar and mutually exclusive formational characteristics of signs have been identified (Doherty, 1985, p 111).

Taction refers to touch. Touch signs are those characterised by one of the signer's hands touching his or her other hand or another part of the body (Nietupski & Hamre-Nietupski, 1979, p 119). "Happy" and "cry" are touch signs. "Car" is a non-touch sign. Research has suggested that touch signs are generally easier to learn than non-touch signs (Doherty, 1985; Doherty & Lloyd, 1983; Dunn, 1979; Fouts, 1972; Kohl, 1981; Stremel-Campbell et al, 1977).

Symmetry pertains to the hand shape and movement requirements of two-handed signs. Symmetrical signs require identical hand shapes and identical or reciprocal movements by the two hands, whereas asymmetrical signs require different hand shapes and/or different movements (Doherty, p 113). "Bicycle" and "push" are symmetrical signs. "Biscuit" is an asymmetrical sign. Symmetrical signs are learned significantly faster than assymetrical signs (Bornstein & Jordan, 1982; Hamre-Nietsupski et al, 1977; Kiernan, 1984; Kiernan & Bowler, 1982), and symmetry is a strong facilitative factor in sign learning (Kohl, 1981).

Handedness refers to the number of hands used in the sign's production (Luftig, 1984, p 195). "Pour" is a one-handed sign. "Basin" is a two-handed sign. Research findings on this aspect of acquisition have been inconclusive.

Visibility is determined by whether the signer is able to see the sign as it is being produced. (Luftig, 1984, p 195). "Toilet" is a visible sign. "Telephone" is a non-visible sign.

Duplication is defined by the sign being produced by a number of repetitive hand motions as opposed to the hand motion being produced just once (Luftig, 1984, p 195). "No" and "scissors" are signs that illustrate duplication. "Hello" does not. Little research has been reported on the influence of this factor on acquisition.

Complexity involves signs that require the production of two distinct motor movements as opposed to signs that require only one movement (Doherty, 1985, p 116). "Want" and "fold" are complex signs. "Help" is not.

Fluidity refers to the smooth transition from one hand shape to another during the production of signs that have different beginning and ending hand shapes (Doherty, p 111). Studies of fluidity seek to determine whether signs characterised by the fluid or smooth transition between discrete beginning and ending hand shapes (such as "apron", "take") are easier or more difficult to acquire than single-movement signs (such as "telephone"), although this is a little researched area.

2. Cheremic Classes and Cheremes

The term "chereme" refers to the visible motoric units of sign languages, much as phonemes have represented the distinctive auditory units of spoken languages (Stokoe, 1960). Every sign is characterised by its cheremes (that is, its distinct hand shape, location, movement and palm orientation) (Cooney, 1985, p 12).

Hand shape can be defined as the shape and position of the fingers during sign production (Dennis et al, 1982, p 21). Hand shape appears to be a significant factor in sign learning (Byler, 1985). Easy-to-imitate postures have been learned faster than difficult-to-imitate postures

(Kiernan, 1984). Kiernan's rank ordering of 27 hand postures by their ease of imitation has suggested that the easiest signs to learn are, in rank order, index finger isolation, thumb isolation, spread hand, pincer hand and whole hand. Dunn (1979), an occupational therapist, has suggested an order for ease of production from simple to complex: whole hand, thumb isolation, index finger isolation, little finger isolation and complex signs. Although Dunn's suggestions and Kiernan's findings are compatible, it must be concluded that much more research is needed to further refine existing knowledge regarding the influence of hand shape on sign learning.

Location has been defined by reference to four areas of the body: face, trunk, arm and hand (Shane & Wilbur, 1980, p 333).

Movement has not yet been operationally defined. Scant references in the literature to kinds of movements have included unilateral/bilateral (Dennis et al, 1982); change of hand shape from closed to open and from open to closed, and finger wiggle (Stokoe, 1960); as well as linear, rotate/twist, circular arc, hold and elbow pivot (Supalla, 1978). The influence of movement on sign learning is largely unknown. However, Dunn has offered two suggestions: (a) the hand-to-mouth movement is basic, practised often and therefore perhaps easier to produce; and (b) movement toward the midline of the body is generally easier than movement away from the midline. The hand-to-mouth movement is illustrated by the sign for "eat". The signs for "paper" and "table" illustrate movements toward and away from the midline respectively.

Palm orientation refers to the orientation of the palm(s) during sign production (Battison, 1974). The two basic orientations of palms-up and palms-down are illustrated by the signs for "bus" and "swim". This aspect of sign learning has been under-researched, although Dunn has suggested that signs requiring palms-up orientation are more difficult to acquire than signs requiring palms-down orientation.

3. Cheremic Similarity

Cheremic similarity refers to the degree to which signs look similar because they share cheremes for one or more of the cheremic classes of hand shape, location, movement and palm orientation (Griffith & Robinson, 1980, p 292). Cheremic similarity is illustrated by the sign pairs "chair"/"elevator" and "knife"/"knit".

Clinical observations have tended to support the premise that teaching signs that exhibit cheremic similarity in close succession causes confusion and interferes with learning (Hamre-Nietupski et al, 1977, p 109; Luftig, 1984, p 194; Musselwhite & St Louis, 1982, p 138; Reichle & Keogh, 1985, p 32). Conversely, considerable empirical evidence has pointed to facilitated effects on learning when signs have been distinctly different and more easily discriminated (Fouts, 1972, 1973; Griffith & Robinson, 1980; Griffith, Robinson & Panagos, 1981; McLean & Snyder-McLean, 1978; Stremel-Campbell et al, 1977).

The above findings suggest that signs taught in succession should be distinctly different; that is, they should not exhibit cheremic similarity. It has therefore been recommended that when similar signs are selected for instruction, difficulties can be minimised by postponing the teaching of one of the signs (Blau, 1983, p 219).

4. In-repertoire Motoric Behaviours

In-repertoire motoric behaviours signify that the learner is able to perform the motor movements required to produce a particular sign. That is, the required movements are already within the learner's motoric repertoire.

It has been suggested that signs for which the learner can perform the motor movements should be taught initially, since learners are most apt to imitate behaviours that are already in their repertoires (Blau, 1983, p 218; Reichle et al, 1981 p 50). Fewer errors in sign articulation are also likely to result if the learner is able to perform the specific motor movements required (Dennis et al, 1982, p 20). Dennis et al have summarised the hand (prehension) and arm (unilateral/bilateral) movement patterns used in the production of signs and have suggested ways to assess the learner's ability to produce these patterns during the activities of daily living. An occupational therapist should, of course, be consulted with regard to any motoric assessment and subsequent therapy. The situation could arise that the learner is incapable of producing a specific motor movement required for the production of a sign and is not likely to do so without a great deal of time and energy being expended. It would then be necessary for the special educator, in consultation with the occupational therapist, to consider the feasibility of persisting with the physical therapy that would enable the learner to produce the movement. Instead, this might be the time to consider some other kind of symbol to represent the needed concept, such as a picture, line drawing or Compic symbol (a pictograph prepared from a standardised set distributed in Melbourne, Victoria, by the Compic Development Association for use by people with severe communication impairment). This would be in keeping with the goal of expediting the learner's communicative abilities by whatever means seem appropriate, given the specific vocabulary item to be represented or the nature of the situation.

Referents that the Signs Represent

Concreteness is an important concept to consider here. A distinction that must be made clear is that concreteness does not refer to signs but, rather, to the referents the signs represent. Referents are concrete or abstract; signs are not.

A definition frequently cited is that of Harrell, Bowers and Bacal (1973), quoted by Luftig (1983, p 280). It characterises concrete referents as having corresponding sense data in the phenomenal world, while abstract referents do not. In simpler terms, concrete referents refer to things in the world that can be seen or heard (such as "dog" and "car") and can be easily mentally envisaged (Luftig & Lloyd, 1981, p 49). Abstract referents refer to things in the world that cannot be easily mentally envisaged (such as "bad" and "pretty").

Concreteness has been relatively well researched with normal learners, with deaf learners and with learners having mild developmental delay. Across that spectrum of learning populations, concrete concepts have been shown to be easier to learn than abstract concepts (Luftig, 1982; 1983, p 280). It is evident that individuals with severe or profound developmental delay have not generally been used as subjects (Luftig, 1983, p 280).

Furthermore, while numerous studies have demonstrated a strong relationship between the concreteness of the referents and verbal learning (that is, the learning of word lists and verbal concepts), the influence of concreteness on sign learning has been largely overlooked (Luftig & Lloyd, 1981, p 51). Luftig and Lloyd could find only one study in which the concreteness of the referents was manipulated in sign learning. In that study, by Conlin and Paivio (1975), it was found that high concreteness combined with ease of signing facilitated sign learning with deaf subjects.

It must be concluded that the hypothesis of a facilitative effect for concrete referents in sign learning has not been based on empirical evidence pertaining to the learning of sign language by individuals with severe or profound developmental delay. Rather, it has been based on interpolations of findings from related studies (Luftig, 1982; Luftig & Lloyd, 1981). Further research is needed in this area in order to arrive at a definitive conclusion.

It has also been hypothesised that a relationship may exist between concreteness of the referent and translucency of the sign. Translucency is defined as "a judgement by learners of the degree of relatedness between a sign and its meaning" (Luftig, 1983, p 279). Consider, for example, the high translucency of the signs representing the concrete referents "baby" and "doll" compared to the low translucency of the signs representing the abstract referents "fun" and "super". The interactive effects of concreteness and translucency still need to be investigated (Luftig, 1983, p 284). Research along those lines would further help to clarify the influence of concreteness of the referent on sign learning.

Perceived Relationship between the Sign and Its Referent

1. Iconicity

Iconicity refers to how a sign visually resembles or is reminiscent of some aspect of its referent (Luftig & Lloyd, 1981, p 50). An iconic sign is one that visually resembles the shape, motion or function of its referent to such a degree that the referent can be guessed from the sign alone (that is, it displays transparency); or to the degree that the relationship between the sign and its referent can be perceived when the referent is known (that is, the sign has translucency) (Doherty, 1985, p 116). "Drink", "come" and "listen" are signs that most people would regard as being transparent or guessable. This is because "drink" strongly resembles the action of drinking while "come" and "listen" are synonymous with the generally understood gestures for these actions.

"Clean", "cordial" and "exist" might be regarded as being translucent in that, although the meaning of the sign may not be immediately apparent as is the case with transparent signs, an association between the sign and its referent can be perceived provided that the client/learner is made aware of the association. For instance, with "clean", the client can easily make the association of flicking dirt off the hands. The sign for "cordial" can be perceived as holding and tilting a glass of something. "Exit" is indicated by the fingers of one hand going out from between the fingers of the other hand.

The distinction between transparency and translucency is such that the meaning of transparent signs is guessable from the signs alone because the association between the sign and its referent is known to the client/learner as an outcome of his everyday experiences. The meaning of translucent signs like "cordial", on the other hand, becomes obvious when the association between the sign and its referent is pointed out to the client. It is common teaching practice to show the learner the sign and to explain its meaning at the same time (that is, translucency).

Take, for example, the sign for milk. While the action of milking a cow may be synonymous with "milk" to many of the older generation, it would not be to an urban-dwelling child with intellectual disability living in the '90s. The sign is quite transparent but the context may not be familiar to the child and therefore the association between the sign and its referent may not be easily perceived. Translucency is more potent than transparency in this example.

Further support for translucency being the more important of the two variables of iconicity has come from the realisation that a much greater percentage of signs in sign language are translucent than are transparent. This was found to be the case with American Sign

Language (Bellugi & Klima, 1976; Luftig, Page & Lloyd, 1981), and a cursory view of signs in the *Dictionary of Australasian Signs* suggests that this is also the case with Australasian Sign Language (Jeanes, Reynolds & Coleman, 1989).

It has been reasoned that iconic signs (that is, those that are translucent to the learner) should be easier to learn initially because they demand less of the learner's representational skills — that is, the ability to associate the sign with its referent (Reichle & Keogh, 1985, p 33). This reasoning is in general agreement with findings from empirical research, which have demonstrated faster acquisition for signs that are iconic (translucent signs as opposed to signs that are not translucent, that is, opaque) (Griffith & Robinson, 1980; Kohl, Karlan & Heal, 1979; Konstantareas, Oxman & Webster, 1978; Luftig, 1983; McLean & Snyder-McLean, 1978).

2. Conceptual Similarity

Conceptual similarity has yet to be defined. However, Doherty (1985, p 118) has assumed from the literature that it refers to either conceptual similarity between two meanings in the same class (such as "pants", "shirt") or between two meanings that share a hierarchical relationship (such as "milk", "drink").

Although no empirical data are available, observational data alone have appeared to support a strategy of choosing conceptually dissimilar signs for learning within the same training session Signs representing referents that are conceptually related have been observed to cause considerable confusion when they have been taught in fairly close succession (Blau, 1983, p 219; Fouts, 1972, 1973; Stremel-Campbell et al, 1977, p 346).

Additionally, children with developmental delay have been seen to experience even more confusion if signs that are conceptually similar have also exhibited cheremic similarity (Byler, 1985, p 111; Stremel-Campbell et al, 1977, p 345). The sign pairs "apple"/"orange" and "wash"/"soap" exhibit both conceptual and cheremic similarity, and it is apparent how easily the signs in each pair could be confused for one another.

Summary

It is apparent from the previous discussion that, while it has been hypothesised that many variables involved in the physical production and visual comprehension of signs are an influence on the ease of sign learning, only the influence of a few has been substantiated by empirical research. Those variables that have been found to facilitate sign learning include taction, symmetry, translucency, in-repertoire motoric behaviours, cheremic dissimilarity (empirical support) and conceptual dissimilarity (strong observational support) when signs are taught in close succession. Hand shape does appear to be significant, but it is not yet clear which hand shapes are easier to learn. The probability is that the facilitation of sign learning might be optimised by organising learning on as many of these relevant variables as possible (Luftig, 1982, p 92).

Although the influence of the other variables has not been substantiated, they should not be dismissed as being unimportant to sign learning. Further research may verify many of the hypotheses that so far have been suggested by observational data. Nor should the significance of the observational data be underestimated. In this area of research, where it is extremely difficult to isolate the variables and the subjects vary so greatly in their motoric production and visual comprehension capabilities, observational data do have a contribution to make. Special educators can, by being cognisant of the physical production and visual comprehension variables that are thought to influence sign learning, apply that knowledge when teaching signs to individual learners and thereby contribute to the accumulation of observational data.

Conclusions

This chapter has examined three kinds of knowledge (developmental, functional and motoric) that are important to decision-making when selecting vocabulary items for initial manual sign language programs. In each of the sections pertaining to these knowledge bases, an attempt has been made to highlight and summarise the information that would assist special educators to select a vocabulary. It is still necessary to consider how the three knowledge bases can be integrated to provide an effective holistic approach toward vocabulary item selection.

Functional usefulness of the item for the learner must always be the first consideration, a theme pervading much of the discussion throughout this chapter. While an ecological approach to vocabulary selection will yield many items that are functional for the learner, the special educator may wish to consider some items represented in the developmental data. Of the many helpful suggestions offered by the developmental data, some are sure to be highly functional for the learner. The selection of vocabulary items begins, then, with specifying items that are functional for the learner, whether those items originate from a functional knowledge base (that is by using an ecological inventory in conjunction with the functional strategies) or from a developmental knowledge base (that is, by consulting the developmental data). Blau (1983, p 231) approved of such an approach, stating that the vocabulary selections made on the basis of developmental guidelines should always be evaluated in terms of their functional usefulness for the learner.

The next and last step is to refine the list of vocabulary items, which have been selected for their functionality, in accordance with the findings relating to the motoric constraints on the ease of sign learning (that is, those constraints of physical production and visual comprehension of signs). This two-step process for vocabulary selection has been advocated by Luftig (1983, p 284) and by Nietupski and Hamre-Nietupski (1979, p 284).

This chapter has shown, through its analysis of research findings on vocabulary selection, that the theoretical literature provides a rich source of information to assist special educators. An understanding of the research findings not only can take much of the guesswork out of lexicon planning but also can provide the means to guide the learner toward communication in the most effective and efficient way possible. Selecting vocabulary items for initial manual sign training programs need not be the daunting task it has often been thought to be. Once these items have been selected, the special educator can teach language learners to use these signs in communicative interactions with other people by following the general principles and practices described in Chapter 8 of this book.

References

Alberto, P.A., Garrett, E., Briggs, T. & Unberger, F. (1983). Selection and initiation of a nonvocal communication program for severely handicapped students. *Focus on Exceptional Children 15 (7)*, 1–16.

Ashton-Warner, S. (1971). *Teacher*. New York: Bantam.

Battison, R. (1974). Phonological deletion in American sign language. *Sign Language Studies 5*, 1–19.

Bellugi, U. & Klima, E. (1976). Two faces of sign: Iconic and abstract. In S. Harmad, H. Steklis & J. Lancaster (eds), *The origins and evaluation of language and speech*. New York: Annals of the New York Academy of Arts and Sciences.

Bernstein, D.K. & Tiegerman, E. (1989). Language and communication disorders in children (2nd edn). Columbus: Charles E. Merrill.

Blau, A.F. (1983). Vocabulary selection in augmentative communication: Where do we begin? In H. Winitz (ed.), *Treating language disorders: For clinicians by clinicians*. Baltimore: University Park Press.

Bloom, L. (1970). *Language development: Form and function in emerging grammars*. Cambridge, Mass.: MIT Press.

Bloom, L. (1973). *One word at a time: The use of single-word utterances before syntax*. The Hague: Mouton.

Bloom, L., Miller, P. & Hood, L. (1978). Variations and reduction as aspects of competence in language development. In L. Bloom (ed.), *Readings in language development*. New York: John Wiley & Sons.

Bloomberg, K. & Johnson, H. (1991). *Communication without speech*. Melbourne: A.C.E.R.

Bochner, S., Price, P. & Salamon, L. (1988). *Learning to talk: A programme for helping language-delayed children acquire early communication skills*. Sydney: Macquarie University.

Bornstein, H. & Jordan, I.K. (1982). *The relationship between sign characteristics and understandability of simpler sign forms*. Paper presented at the VIth Congress of the International Association for the Scientific Study of Mental Deficiency, Toronto.

Bottorf, L. & DePape, D. (1982). Initiating communication systems for severely speech-impaired persons. *Topics in Language Disorders 2*, 55–71.

Bowerman, M. (1978). Semantic and syntactic development: A review of what, when, and how in language acquisition. In R.L. Schiefelbusch (ed.), *Bases of language intervention*. Baltimore: University Park Press.

Brown, R. (1973). *A first language: The early steps*. London: George Allen & Unwin Ltd.

Brown, L., Nietupski, J. & Hamre-Nietupski, S. (1976). The criterion of ultimate functioning and public school services for severely handicapped students. In M.A. Thomas (ed.), *Hey don't forget about me: Education's investment in the severely, profoundly and multiply handicapped*. Reston: Council for Exceptional Children.

Bryen, D.N., Goldman, A.S. & Quinlisk-Gill, S. (1988). Sign language with students with severe/profound mental retardation: How effective is it? *Education and Training in Mental Retardation 23 (2)*, 129–37.

Bryen, D.N. & Joyce, D.G. (1985). Language intervention with the severely handicapped: A decade of research. *Journal of Special Education 19*, 7–39.

Byler, J.K. (1985). The Makaton Vocabulary: An analysis based on recent research. *British Journal of Special Education 12 (3)*, 109–16.

Carlson, F. (1981). A format for selecting vocabulary for the nonspeaking child. *Language, Speech and Hearing Services in Schools 12*, 240–45.

Clarke, S., Remington, B. & Light, P. (1986). An evaluation of the relationship between receptive speech skills and expressive signing. *Journal of Applied Behavior Analysis 19*, 231–39.

Cole, M.L. & Cole, J.T. (1981). *Effective intervention with the language impaired child*. Rockville: Aspen Systems Corporation.

Conlin, D. & Paivio, A. (1975). The associative learning of the deaf: The effects of word imagery and signability. *Memory and Cognition 3*, 335–40.

Cooney, A. (1985). Nonverbal communication systems and their use with mentally retarded people. In A.F. Ashman & R.S. Laura (eds), *The education and training of the mentally retarded*. Sydney: Croom Helm.

Dayan, M., Harper, B., Molloy, J.S. & Witt, B.T. (1977). *Communication for the severely and profoundly handicapped*. Denver: Love Publishing Co.

Dennis, R., Reichle, J., Williams, W. & Vogelsberg, R.T. (1982). Motoric factors influencing the selection of vocabulary for sign production programs. *Teaching Association for the Severely Handicapped Journal 7 (1)*, 20–32.

Doherty, J.E. (1985). The effects of sign characteristics on sign acquisition and retention: An integrative review of the literature. *Augmentative and Alternative Communication 1*, 108–21.

Doherty, J. & Lloyd, L. (1983). *Effects of production mode, translucency, and manuality on sign acquisition by retarded adults*. Unpublished manuscript. Dallas: American Association on Mental Deficiency.

Duchan, J.F. (1988). Language assessment: The pragmatics revolution. In R.C. Naremore (ed.), *Language science: Recent advances*. San Diego: College Hill Press.

Dunn, M.L. (1979). *Analysis of the motor component of imitative sign production*. A miniseminar presented at the American Speech-Language-Hearing Association Convention, Atlanta. In C.R. Musselwhite & K.W. St Louis (1982). *Communication programming for the severely handicapped: Vocal and non-vocal strategies*. Houston: College Hill Press.

Fouts, R. (1972). Use of guidance in teaching sign language to a chimpanzee (Pan troglodytes). *Journal of Comparative and Physiological Psychology 80*, 515–22.

Fouts, R. (1973). Acquisition and testing of gestural signs in four young chimpanzees. *Science 180*, 978–80.

Fristoe, M. & Lloyd, L.L. (1979). Sign vocabularies used in manual communication training with persons having severe communication impairment. *American Association for the Education of the Severely/Profoundly Handicapped Review 4*, 364–73.

Fristoe, M. & Lloyd, L.L. (1980). Planning an initial expressive sign lexicon for persons with severe communication impairment. *Journal of Speech and Hearing Disorders 45*, 170–80.

Gillham, B. (1979). *The first words language programme*. Beaconsfield, Surrey: George Allen & Unwin.

Granville Work Preparation Centre and the Research and Development Project (1980). *The social skills training package*. Sydney: Macquarie University.

Griffith, P.L. & Robinson, J.H. (1980). Influence of iconicity and phonological similarity on sign learning by mentally retarded children. *American Journal of Mental Deficiency 85*, 291–98.

Griffith, P.L., Robinson, J.H. & Panagos, J.M. (1981). Perception of iconicity in American Sign Language by hearing and deaf subjects. *Journal of Speech and Hearing Disorders 46*, 388–97.

Hamre-Nietupski, S., Stoll, A., Holtz, K., Fullerton, P., Ryan-Flottum, M. & Brown, L. (1977). Curricular strategies for teaching selected nonverbal communication skills to nonverbal and verbal severely handicapped students. In Madison Metropolitan School District, *Curricular strategies for teaching functional object use, nonverbal communication, problem solving, and mealtime skills to severely handicapped students* (vol. VII). Madison: Department of Specialized Educational Services, Madison Metropolitan School District.

Harrell, M., Bowers, J.W. & Bacal, J.P. (1973). Another stab at meaning: Concreteness and conventionality. *Speech Nonographs 40*, 199–207.

Holland, A. (1975). Language therapy for children: Some thoughts on context and content. *Journal of Speech and Hearing Disorders 40*, 514–23.

Jeanes, R.C., Reynolds, B.E. & Coleman, B.C. (1989). *Dictionary of Australasian signs* (2nd edn). Brunswick, Vic.: Glove Press Pty Ltd.

Johnson, H. (1986). Learning day by day and where to begin. In B. Dredge & C. Crosthwaite (eds), *Communication without speech*. Melbourne: Commonwealth Schools Commission.

Jones, T.W. (1980). Is it necessary to decide whether to use a nonoral communication system with retarded children? *Education and Training of the Mentally Retarded 15*, 157–60.

Kaiser, A.P., Alpert, C.L., & Warren, S.F. (1987). Teaching functional language: Strategies for language intervention. In M.E. Snell (ed.), *Systematic instruction of persons with severe handicaps* (3rd edn). Columbus: Charles E. Merrill.

Karlan, G.R. & Lloyd, L.L. (1983). Considerations in the planning of communication intervention: Selecting a lexicon. *Teaching Association for the Severely Handicapped 8*, 13–25.

Keogh, W.J. & Reichle, J. (1982). *Teaching 'want'*. Paper presented at the national conference of the Association for the Severely Handicapped, Denver.

Keogh, W.J. & Reichle, J. (1985). Communication intervention for the 'difficult-to-teach' severely handicapped. In S.F. Warren & A.K. Rogers-Warren (eds), *Teaching functional language: Generalization and maintenance of language skills*. Baltimore: University Park Press.

Kiernan, C. (1984). The imitation and learning of hand postures. In J.M. Berg (ed.), *Perspective and progress in mental retardation* (vol. 1) Baltimore: University Park Press.

Kiernan, C.C. & Bowler, D.M. (1982). *The imitation and learning of hand postures by normal and mentally handicapped children*. Paper presented at the VIth Congress of the International Association for the Scientific Study of Mental Deficiency, Toronto.

Kiernan, C.C., Reid, B. & Goldbart, J. (1987). *Foundations of communication and language: Course manual*. Manchester: Manchester University Press.

Kohl, F.L. (1981). Effects of the motoric requirements on the acquisition of manual sign responses by severely handicapped students. *American Journal of Mental Deficiency 85*, 396–403.

Kohl, F.L., Karlan, G.R. & Heal, L.W. (1979). Effects of pairing manual signs with verbal cues upon the acquisition of instruction-following behaviours and the generalization to expressive language with severely handicapped students. *American Association for the Education of the Severely/Profoundly Handicapped Review 4*, 291–300.

Konstantareas, M., Oxman, J. & Webster, C.D. (1978). Iconicity: Effects on the acquisition of sign language by autistic and other severely dysfunctional children. In P. Siple (ed.), *Understanding language through sign language research*. New York: Academic Press.

Kopchick, G.A. & Lloyd, L.L. (1976). Total communication for the severely language impaired: A 24-hour approach. In L.L. Lloyd (ed.), *Communication assessment and intervention strategies*. Baltimore: University Park Press.

Lahey, M. & Bloom, L. (1977). Planning a first lexicon: Which words to teach first. *Journal of Speech and Hearing Disorders 42*, 340–50.

Leeming, K., Swann, W., Coupe, J. & Mittler, P. (1979). *Teaching language and communication to the mentally handicapped*. London: Evans/Methuen Educational.

Lombardino, L.J., Willems, S. & MacDonald, J.D. (1981). Critical considerations in total communication and an environmental intervention model for the developmentally delayed. *Exceptional Children 47*, 455–61.

Lucas, E.V. (1980). *Semantic and pragmatic language disorders: Assessment and remediation*. Rockville: Aspen Systems Corporation.

Luftig, R.L. (1982). Increasing probability of sign language learning by severely mentally retarded individuals: A discussion of learner, sign production, and linguistic variables. *Applied Research in Mental Retardation 3*, 81–97.

Luftig, R.L. (1983). Translucency of sign and concreteness of gloss in the manual sign learning of moderately/severely mentally retarded students. *American Journal of Mental Deficiency 88 (3)*, 279–86.

Luftig, R.L. (1984). An analysis of initial sign lexicons as a function of eight learnability variables. *Journal of the Association for Persons with Severe Handicaps 9 (3)*, 193–200.

Luftig, R.L. & Lloyd, L.L. (1981). Manual sign translucency and referential concreteness in the learning of sign. *Sign Language Studies 30*, 49–60.

Luftig, R.L., Page, J. & Lloyd, L. (1981). *Translucency of manual signs*. Unpublished manuscript. W. Lafayette: Purdue University.

McCormick, L.M. (1990). Sequence of language and communication development. In L.M. McCormick & R.L. Schiefelbusch (eds), *Early language intervention* (2nd edn). Columbus: Charles E. Merrill.

McCormick, L. & Goldman, R. (1984). Designing an optimal learning program. In L. McCormick & R.L. Schiefelbusch (eds), *Early language intervention*. Columbus: Charles E. Merrill.

McCormick, L.M. & Schiefelbusch, R.L. (1990). An introduction to language intervention. In L.M. McCormick & R.L. Schiefelbusch (eds), *Early language intervention* (2nd edn). Columbus: Charles E. Merrill.

McDonald, J.D. (1982). Communication strategies for language intervention. In D.P. McClowry, A.M. Guildford & S.O. Richardson (eds), *Infant communication: Development, assessment and intervention*. New York: Grune & Stratton.

McLean, J.E. & Snyder-McLean, L.K. (1978). *Transactional approach to early language training*. Columbus: Charles E. Merrill.

McLean, J.E. & Snyder-McLean, L.K. (1987). Form and function of communicative behaviour among persons with severe developmental disabilities. *Australia and New Zealand Journal of Developmental Disabilities 13 (2)*, 83–98.

Meyers, L.S., Anderson, C. & Liddicoat, M. (1984). Perceived communication needs of developmentally delayed nonspeaking children. *The Psychology Record 34*, 55–68.

Miller, J. & Allaire, J. (1987). Augmentative communication. In M.E. Snell (ed.), *Systematic instruction of persons with severe handicaps*. Columbus: Charles E. Merrill.

Moerk, E.L. (1977). *Pragmatic and semantic aspects of early language development*. Baltimore: University Park Press.

Montgomery, J.K. (1986). Communication: Application from research in nonverbal studies. *Remedial and Special Education 7 (2)*, 32–8.

Moores, D.F. (1974). Nonvocal systems of verbal behaviour. In R.L. Schiefelbusch & L.L. Lloyd (eds), *Language perspectives: Acquisition, retardation, and intervention*. Baltimore: University Park Press.

Musselwhite, C.R. & St Louis, K.W. (1982). *Communication programming for the severely handicapped: Vocal and non-vocal strategies*. Houston: College Hill Press.

Nelson, K. (1973). Some evidence for the cognitive primacy of categorization and its functional basis. *Merrill-Palmer Quarterly 19*, 21–39.

Nietupski, J. & Hamre-Nietupski, S. (1977). Nonverbal communication and severely handicapped students: A review of selected literature. In L. Brown, J. Nietupski, S. Lyon, S. Hamre-Nietupski, T. Crowner & L. Gruenewald (eds), *Curricular strategies for teaching functional object use, nonverbal communication, problem solving, and mealtime skills to severely handicapped students*. Madison: Madison Metropolitan School District.

Nietupski, J. & Hamre-Nietupski, S. (1979). Teaching auxiliary communication skills to severely handicapped students. *American Association for the Education of the Severely/Profoundly Handicapped Review 4 (2)*, 107–24.

Owens, R. & House, L. (1984). Decision making processes in augmentative communication. *Journal of Speech and Hearing Disorders 49*, 18–25.

Porter, P.B. (1987). Language vs. communication in training for augmentative communication use. In S.M. Attermeier (ed.), *Augmentative communication: Clinical issues*. New York: The Haworth Press.

Poulton, K.T. & Algozzine, B. (1980). Manual communication and mental retardation: A review of research and implications. *American Journal of Mental Deficiency 85 (2)*, 145–52.

Rees, N. (1978). Pragmatics of language: Applications to normal and disordered language development. In R.L. Schiefelbusch (ed.), *Basis of language intervention*. Baltimore: University Park Press.

Reichle, J. & Karlan, G. (1985). The selection of an augmentative system in communication intervention: A critique of decision rules. *Journal of the Association for Persons with Severe Handicaps 10*, 146–56.

Reichle, J. & Keogh, W.J. (1985). Communication intervention: A selection review of what, when, and how to teach. In S.F. Warren & A.K. Rogers-Warren (eds) *Teaching functional language: Generalization and maintenance of language skills*. Baltimore: University Park Press.

Reichle, J., Williams, W. & Ryan, S. (1981). Selecting signs for the formulating of an augmentative communication modality. *Teaching Association for the Severely Handicapped Journal 6*, 48–54.

Romski, M.A., Sevcik, M.A. & Ellis Joyner, S. (1984). Nonspeech communication systems: Implications for language intervention with mentally retarded children. *Topics in Language Disorders 5*, 66–81.

Russell, M. (1984). Assessment and intervention issues with the non-speaking child. *Exceptional Children 51 (1)*, 64–71.

Schaeffer, B. (1980a). Teaching signed speech to non-verbal children: Theory and method. *Sign Language Studies 26*, 29–63.

Schaeffer, B. (1980b). Spontaneous language through signed speech. In R.L. Schiefelbusch (ed.), *Nonspeech language and communication: Analysis and intervention*. Baltimore: University Park Press.

Scheuerman, N., Baumgart, D., Sipsma, K. & Brown, L. (1976). Toward the development of a curriculum for teaching nonverbal communication skills to severely handicapped students: Teaching basic tracking, scanning, and selection skills. In N. Scheuerman, L. Brown & T. Crowner (eds), *Toward an integrated therapy model for teaching motor, tracking and scanning skills to severely handicapped students* (Vol. VI). Madison: Madison Metropolitan School District.

Schlesinger, I.M. (1971). Production of utterances and language acquisition. In D. Slobin (ed.), *The ontogenesis of grammar*. New York: Academic Press.

Shane, H.C. & Wilbur, R. (1980). Potential for expressive signing based on motor control. *Journal of Sign Language Studies 29*, 331–47.

Siegel-Causey, E. & Guess, D. (1989). *Enhancing nonsymbolic communication interactions among learners with severe disabilities*. Baltimore: Paul H. Brookes.

Silverman, F.H. (1980). *Communication for the speechless*. Englewood Cliffs, NJ: Prentice-Hall.

Stokoe, W. (1960). Sign language structure. *Studies in linguistics: Occasional papers* (No. 8). Buffalo, NY: University of Buffalo Press.

Stremel-Campbell, K., Cantrell, D. & Halle, J. (1977). Manual signing as a language system and as a speech initiator for the non-verbal severely handicapped student. In E. Sontag, J. Smith & N. Certo (eds), *Educational programming for the severely and profoundly handicapped*. Reston, V: Division on Mental Retardation, Council for Exceptional Children.

Supalla, T. (1978). *Morphology of verbs of motion and location in ASL*. Paper presented at the National Symposium on Sign Language Research and Teaching, San Diego.

Walker, M. (1984). *The revised Makaton Vocabulary*. In M. Walker & A. Cooney, The revised Makaton Vocabulary (Australian version). Unpublished manuscript. Newcastle, NSW: Makaton Vocabulary Development Project, Australian Resource Unit, Newcastle College of Advanced Education.

Warren, S.F. & Rogers-Warren, A. (1985). Teaching functional language: An introduction. In S.F. Warren and A.K. Rogers-Warren (eds), *Teaching functional language: Generalization and maintenance of language skills*. Baltimore: University Park Press.

Wells, G. (1981). Language as interaction. In G. Wells (ed.), *Learning through interaction: The study of language development*. Cambridge: Cambridge University Press.

Winitz, H. (1983). Use and abuse of the developmental approach. In H. Winitz (ed.), *Treating language disorders: For clinicians by clinicians*. Baltimore: University Park Press.

Wolfensberger, W. (1972). *The principle of normalization in human services*. Toronto: National Institute of Mental Retardation.

Wood, B.S. (1981). *Children and communication: Verbal and nonverbal language development* (2nd edn). Englewood Cliffs, NJ: Prentice-Hall.

Woolman, D.H. (1974). A presymbolic training program. In R.L. Schiefelbusch & L.L. Lloyd (eds), *Language perspectives: Acquisition, retardation, and intervention*. Baltimore: University Park Press.

Yoder, D. & Kraat, A. (1983). Intervention issues in nonspeech communication. In J. Miller, D. Yoder & R. Schiefelbusch (eds), *Contemporary issues in language intervention*. Rockville: American Speech-Language-Hearing Association.

Chapter 5

Functional Communication and the Role of Context*

Ken Linfoot
Charles Sturt University-Mitchell
Bathurst, NSW

Over the years there has been a change of focus in research on language development, away from the earlier phonologically based structural approaches (Bloomfield, 1933; Wepman, 1959), the nativistic theories of syntax acquisition (Chomsky, 1957) and the behavioural learning theory explanations (Skinner, 1957; Staats, 1968). More recent theories have emphasised psycholinguistic and sociolinguistic bases for, or "transactional" explanations of, language learning. These models, proposed in the late 1970s (Bloom & Lahey, 1978; McLean & Snyder-McLean, 1978), have had considerable impact on research and practice affecting the education of children with intellectual disabilities. "Pragmatics" is the term used for the system of rules describing the way children learn to use language in a variety of contexts to achieve their communicative purposes (Bates, 1976) and is derived from theory on "speech acts" (Searle, 1969), where utterances are viewed in terms of the speaker's purpose in performing them. Along with phonology, semantics and syntax dimensions of linguistic behaviour, pragmatics is considered to be an important focus of intervention attempting to assist affected individuals to overcome problems of communication skill development.

Research describing young children's development of pragmatics skills has included normally developing children (Bates, 1976; Dore, 1974; Halliday, 1975) and children with communication difficulties (such as McLean, McLean, Brady & Etter, 1991; Miller, in press;

*An earlier version of this paper was presented in Dublin to the conference of the International Association for the Scientific Study of Mental Deficiency, 1988.

Wetherby & Prutting, 1984). However, it is for children with intellectual disability that research interest in the *uses* of communication by young children (pragmatics) has particular relevance. For children with intellectual disabilities, O'Connor and Hermelin (1962) had noted difficulties in "using words, even when these were available (known) to them" and later writers have drawn attention to delays in language use beyond those anticipated from measures of cognitive development (Cardosa-Martens, Mervis & Mervis, 1985; Miller, in press). Thus, an apparent reluctance to use their available language system may be identified as part of the particular communication difficulty experienced by many children with severe intellectual disability.

All of this suggests that the transactional models of communication development may be helpful in better understanding the problems of children with intellectual disabilities in actually getting to *use* communication forms for interactive purposes. Influenced by earlier theoretical models, facilitators of a child's emerging communicative behaviour might have considered developing such skills as vocabulary knowledge, sentence length, articulation and so on. However, using the transactional model, practitioners will focus more clearly on the uses, or communicative functions, that the language or other behaviour serves for the child. In addition, the moderating variables present, both within the child (such as age, gender, developmental skill levels, communication mode) and within the setting (such as activity type, number and relationship to child of the people present) are possible sources of influence on the ways in which communicative behaviour develops, or can be facilitated.

The present chapter reviews a number of studies that have attempted to identify pragmatic features of the communicative behaviour of this population. This review does show that there are contextual features that appear to influence the communicative functions of children with intellectual disability. The remaining and major part of this chapter describes an investigation of the influence of variations in the lesson context and teaching arrangements within special classrooms, on the communicative behaviour of children with severe intellectual disability. Data produced in this study may have some implications for teachers of this population as they seek to increase the *functional* communication abilities of children who, in the past, have often shown extreme reluctance to engage in communication.

Research Review

Miller (1981) distinguished four levels at which pragmatic functions may be performed by speakers. These include utterance-level functions relevant to the communicative act itself, such as informing, labelling and so on. Secondly, discourse-level functions relating to the conversational or discourse role (answering and initiating) of the communicative act can also be identified. Thirdly, other language at this level may relate to broader discourse functions such as opening a conversation, taking one's turn and so on. Finally, a social level of pragmatic functions can be identified, where reference is needed to the context of the social interaction between speaker and listener. Thus, to be polite or to be persuasive or to portray leadership or dominance may be pragmatic functions identified at this social level (Miller, 1981, pp 112–13).

Table 5-1: Pragmatic functions of children with intellectual disability.

Author(s)		N	Chronological age	Sample	Outcome
Cirrin & Rowland (1985)		15	10 to 18 yrs	Severe/profound retardation; non-verbal	Differences in function usage depending on rate of communication
Coggins & Carpenter (1980)		16	15 to 16 mths	Normally developing infants	Request object, comment, request action most often used
Harris (1984)		6	5 & 9/12 to 10 & 4/12 years	Severe retardation; pre-verbal to Brown Stage I	More spontaneity and initiations in group than 1-to-1 lessons
Light, Collier & Parnes (1985)		8	4 and 6 years	Physically disabled; non-vocal	More communication functions in elicited contexts than play contexts
Owens & MacDonald (1982)		12	20 to 89 mths	Down syndrome (6); non-delayed (6)	Practising only difference between groups for pragmatic function usage
Owings, McManus & Scherer (1981)		1	28 yrs	Moderately retarded	Variations in functions used, depending on speaker and setting
Rowland (1990)	*Study 1*	6	3 to 6 yrs	Deaf/blind; multiple cognitive and motor impairments	Most communication opportunities offered by teachers in group activities, least in language programs
	Study 2	14	3 to 15 yrs	As above	Teachers adapted communication opportunities to available sensory modalities of subjects
Wetherby & Prutting (1984)		8	6 to 12 yrs (E)	Autistic group	Limited range of pragmatic functions for autistic group
			1 to 2 yrs (C)	Mean Length of Utterance matched normals	

The following studies involve pragmatic functions at the utterance level in the main, and also give some attention to discourse roles of communicative behaviour. A summary of the studies reviewed, showing their major characteristics, appears in Table 5-1.

Cirrin and Rowland (1985) described the communicative functions shown by a sample of non-verbal 10- to 18-year-old residents of a state institution. Forty minutes of videotape were collected for each individual with a known adult in "a series of activities . . . devised to promote dyadic interaction and social communication" (p 53).

A coding scheme for pragmatic functions, derived from the work of Chapman (1981), Coggins and Carpenter (1980) and Dore (1974), was used to classify "utterance"-level functions, although these children only used non-verbal communicative behaviour.

Request object, request action and *direct attention to object* were the most frequently used functions, while *pointing* (26% of occurrences), *signing* (18%), *physical contact* (17%) and *extending an object* (16%) were the most frequently used means of communication.

For low-frequency communicators, pragmatic functions were mainly limited to "primary" goals of *request object, request action* and *protest.* High-frequency communicators engaged in more shared activities with a partner, using functions such as *direct attention to object, to action* and *to communicate.*

These data were interpreted by the authors as suggesting a possible developmental sequence of communicative behaviours in this population. However, since the context in which observations are made may influence the nature of communicative behaviour, such generalisations should probably be made only after observations in a variety of contexts.

Harris (1984) investigated the effects of different types of teaching or lesson activities upon the nature of the interactions between teachers and children with severe intellectual disabilities. Ten-minute video recordings were made of children in each of two classes, for both one-to-one and group lessons. Individual and group lessons were contrasted.

Teacher questioning was found to be more controlling and structuring of children's responses in the individual teaching sessions, while the proportion of teacher questions decreased considerably when teachers worked with groups instead of individuals (p 20). Children's utterances were analysed as *answers* or *initiations,* which were further divided into whether or not they were spontaneous, and were also examined for appropriateness.

The results showed that the proportions of children's answering utterances decreased markedly from individual to group sessions, while spontaneous utterances were most frequent in group settings.

A higher proportion of utterances in group sessions than in individual sessions was observed to be appropriate. These findings followed a similar pattern for all class members (p 22).

This study has important implications for research into the pragmatic functions of communication with children in school settings. It draws attention to the effects of the particular class activities, or lesson contexts, upon children's opportunities for spontaneous interactions involving the use of initiations, or conversational openers.

Harris claimed that initiation is the discourse function that allows the child to judge the effect and appropriateness of the original intention in the light of a conversational partner's subsequent response (p 23). Thus, contexts that encourage the use of this pragmatic function are important in communication skill development. Harris has shown that there are lesson activities for language-delayed children, where opportunities can be made for intervention procedures based on an "interactional view of language and communication" (p 24).

Owens and MacDonald (1982) compared Stage I and Stage III speech samples (Brown, 1973) from Down syndrome (developmentally delayed) and non-delayed children. Data analysis included the identification of 100 utterances for each child, drawn from observations made of the children in free-play interactions with their mothers in their own homes.

Overall, a consistent pattern in the use of the functions, termed "illocutionary acts" in this study, was noted for Down syndrome and non-delayed children and at each of Stages I and III.

Answering was the most frequently used communicative function, at 26.7% of occurrences overall and as high as 34.3% for the Stage III Down syndrome children. *Declare, reply, suggest* (command, demand or request) and *practise* had "moderate overall frequencies" (p 506) at 17.8 to 12.8%, while the *question* and *name* categories were used for 8.1 and 5.8% of acts overall. Owens and MacDonald report similar rank ordering of illocutionary acts, with the exception of *practise,* across the subject groups (p 507).

This seems to be somewhat at odds with research by Halliday (1975) examining the communicative behaviour of his own infant son. Halliday reported the simultaneous emergence of *instrumental, regulatory, interactional* and *personal* functions. Similarly, the speech acts of the children "M" and "J" reported by Dore (1973) were rather different from the Owens and MacDonald study. "*Imitating words*" was the most commonly used function in Dore's sample, with "*labelling* items and action patterns" the next most frequently used. "*Answering* a question" was at best a middle-order function for those children (p 123).

These differences may of course reflect different methodologies used by studies to observe children's pragmatic behaviour but may also be explained by differences between the contexts in which the observed children were communicating. It does appear that differences between setting contexts, as well as between the precise definitions of communicative functions, will render comparisons of the results of such experimental studies very difficult.

Contextual effects were considered in a study by Owings, McManus and Scherer (1981). The contexts studied included situations involving (1) two adult residents of an institution; (2) an adult resident talking to a counsellor; and (3) an adult resident "talking to himself" (p 120). The subject of the study was a 28-year-old male classified as "moderately retarded", who was a resident of a state institution (p 120).

Analysis of the speaker's communication in the three settings indicated the speaker's sensitivity to the social and communicative demands of the settings. *Questions to counsellor* and *to peer* represented 29 and 25% of the speaker's utterances, but only 6% of utterances were *questions to self*. *Information-giving* comprised 36% of utterances *to counsellor*, but only 18% of utterances *to peer*, where it may not have been as socially appropriate. Similarly, *commands to peer* and *to self* represented 17 and 18% of utterances in those settings, but only 4% of utterances were *commands to counsellor*, to whom it would be inappropriate for residents to address a command (p 126).

A more comprehensive investigation of the communicative functions used by people with disabilities would be a useful basis for designing intervention strategies in educational and residential settings for the care and development of this population.

Rowland (1990) reported two studies which were concerned with different aspects of the opportunities for communication that are created by teachers of children with dual sensory and multiple cognitive and motor impairments. In the first of these, data were collected from six children aged from three to six years throughout the full day of their attendance at school over a five-week period. Results of these observations showed that most "cues for communication" were offered by teachers and others in the classroom during activities that were food-related or associated with departure from school, toileting, group activities or language lessons, although the latter activities occupied just 3% of the school day. Rowland's second study then demonstrated that a strong relationship existed, across subjects, between opportunities for communication and the children's actual communicative behaviour. Combining results from these two studies, one can see that children's communicative behaviour, while dependent on the frequency of environmental cues or opportunities for communication, is also influenced by the naturally occurring daily activities in classrooms, the language-learning "milieu" described by Hart and Risley (1968) and Hart and Rogers-Warren (1978).

Finally, Light, Collier and Parnes (1985) compared the range of "communicative functions produced by nonspeaking, physically disabled children in a free play context with their primary caregivers, to those within [an] eliciting context with a clinician". The children were aged four to six years, were non-vocal, had normal receptive language skills and were accustomed to using communication boards. McCormick and Schiefelbusch (1990, p 436) describe a communication board as "any type of flat surface on which written or drawn symbols (or even miniature objects) can be displayed".

In the free play with caregiver setting, the most commonly used functions involved responding to the caregiver in some way. Children used the *confirmation/denial* function for 39% of their utterances and *provision of information* for 18.4%. *Requesting objects* or *action* was the only other widely used function at 10.1%. Interestingly, the caregivers' communicative behaviour in this setting largely involved *requesting information* or *clarification of their children's utterances* (45.1%), or *providing information* (24.6%).

In the eliciting context with a clinician, additional communicative functions were observed in the children. These included *social routines* (greetings, closings) and *requests for attention, clarification* and *information* (p 104).

The authors acknowledged that the free-play context might not have created the need for the children to use the wider variety of functions. Or, the caregivers' actions in *requesting information* of the children for much of the time may have reduced their opportunity to use many of the other functions. Additionally, this study presented a difficulty as children and their communication partners needed to be skilled in the use of communication boards. It could be expected that clinicians would be more effective users of such aids than children's own parent-caregivers.

Associated with this problem is the observation of Calculator and Dollaghan (1982), reported by Light et al (p 105), that communication boards provide large symbol vocabularies which enable propositional statements to be made but usually offer no means for users to mark the communicative intents of their utterances. In view of recent advocacy of the use of systems of augmented communication for non-vocal individuals, this concern may need to be carefully addressed when fitting individuals with such systems.

Perhaps the most striking outcome of these studies is the way in which particular observation contexts were associated with the range of pragmatic functions used by the subjects. While language- and developmentally-delayed children may indeed need to master the same communicative functions as non-delayed children, these studies have shown that circumstances often exist in these children's environments (such as institutionalisation, motor control difficulties, the need to use augmented communication systems) that can result in unusual interaction styles with caregivers and that can have significant contextual effects on children's pragmatic communication skills. While a number of studies have shown that language-delayed children often can employ normal pragmatic skills (Harris, 1984; Owens & MacDonald, 1982), others have shown that they frequently use limited pragmatic functions (Cirrin & Rowland, 1985; Wetherby & Prutting, 1984).

In view of the apparent influence of context, the study reported below was designed to examine the effects of variations in classroom lesson contexts on a broad range of types of children's communicative behaviour. The functions of communicative acts were identified as dependent variables, while lesson context (degree of teacher-structuring) was the manipulated variable. The developmental level of children in the classrooms was also identified as a moderator variable.

Methodology

Research Design

A naturalistic observation study was conducted with children from two classrooms of a school attached to a large residential institution providing care for children with severe intellectual disability.

Teaching-context differences were defined in terms of changes in the way the teacher had arranged the lesson format, ranging from one with a high degree of teacher structuring, to one with less, and finally to a lesson format with little teacher structuring of children's responses at all. High-structure lessons (Context 1) consisted of the morning talk, where children were seated in a semicircle in front of the teacher at the start of the school day and exchanged morning greetings, discussed classroom or school news and were addressed individually by the teacher. Medium-structure lessons (Context 2) involved craft or other group activities, where the eight children in the class were seated around a large table and were engaged in an activity such as making Christmas decorations, preparing a cake mixture, or other craft or cooking activities. This group work was directed by the teacher, but there was opportunity for children to initiate interactions with each other or with the teacher. Low-structure lessons (Context 3) were "free-play" activities, where toys, games, old clothes or other play items were placed around the classroom, allowing children to make their own decisions about activity or communication. The teacher's only involvement was to respond to

Table 5-2: Research design.

Class	Time (weeks)			
	1	9 Observations	17 Observations	25 Observations
1	Pilot study	C1 C2 C3	C1 C2 C3	C1 C2 C3
2	Pilot study	C1 C2 C3	C1 C2 C3	C1 C2 C3

Code: C1, C2 and C3 = Observations conducted in Contexts 1, 2 and 3.
The order in which observations were made in each context was determined randomly for each child.

Table 5-3: Sample characteristics.

Child	Age	Sex	Cause and nature of disability	Duration in institution
Class 1				
01	13.9	M	Down syndrome; dwarf; myopic	5 years
02	11.2	M	Hypoglycaemia; epilepsy	4 years
03	11.2	M	Genetic (?); epilepsy	4 years
04	08.1	M	Unknown; epilepsy	4 years
05	09.6	M	Genetic (?)/unknown; secondary autism	4 years
06	12.9	M	Post-natal fever; hypotonic; abnormal EEG; epilepsy	5 years
07	09.9	F	Unknown; microcephaly; epilepsy; hyperkinetic	3 years
08	09.8	M	Unknown; hyperactivity	3 years
Class 2				
09	13.7	F	Unknown, epilepsy	4 years
10	12.8	F	Unknown, epilepsy; abnormal EEG	7 years
11	14.1	M	Tuberous sclerosis; hyperkinetic; epilepsy	7 years
12	11.8	M	Birth asphyxiation	2 years
13	14.8	M	Rubinstein Taby syndrome; dwarfism; psychotic behaviour	9 years
14	11.4	F	Unknown; epilepsy	4 years
15	14.1	M	Down syndrome	7 years
16	14.2	M	Meningitis; dwarfism	5 years

Note: Information on the children's medical conditions was obtained from medical files maintained by the hospital.

children's advances, or to model the use of a particular toy if an uninvolved child was nearby. However, no instruction was given and no controlling moves were made toward children in this setting.

Observations were made on three occasions for each context condition, with two months between each observation period. A pilot study was conducted before the main observation study began. This was a trial of the research design and data collection and analysis procedures. The research design is set out in Table 5-2.

The Sample

The children studied were 12 boys and 4 girls. They met the classification criteria for having an intellectual disability according to

Table 5-4: Formal assessments.

Child	Assessments					
	BSID MA Months	AAMD Indp PR	AAMD Lang PR	AAMD Soc PR	PPVT(L) MA/RS Months	REEL(C) Months
Class 1						
1	<02	04	15	04	25/7	5.5
2	04	BN	05	03	22/2	3.5
3	<02	05	15	02	24/5	8.5
4	>23	39	49	38	26/9	11
5	>23	25	58	21	30/15	22
6	05	04	10	03	BN/0	3
7	02	BN	15	BN	BN/0	4
8	>30	55	60	60	37/26	15
Class 2						
9	06	01	15	01	21/1	6.5
10	NC	20	40	15	23/3	10.5
11	NC	19	19	12	BN/0	8.5
12	NC	50	39	52	26/8	20
13	24	21	42	40	30/15	30
14	04	BN	BN	BN	BN/0	7
15	NC	36	29	41	27/10	20
16	>30	21	40	41	28/12	30

Code: BSID = Bayley Scales of Infant Development
AAMD = AAMD Adaptive Behavior Scale
PPVT(L) = Peabody Picture Vocabulary Test — Form L
REEL(C) = Receptive/Expressive Emergent Language Scale (Combined)
MA = Mental age
Indp Lang Soc = Independence Language Socialisation
RS = Raw score
PR = Percentile rank
BN = Below norms published for score/age
NC = Child did not cooperate in assessment

Grossman (1983). Obvious deficits in adaptive behaviour had resulted in their being institutionalised for most of their lives. All the children had been assessed using the AAMD Adaptive Behavior Scale (ABS) (Nihira et al, 1974) as part of the residential institution procedures. However, intellectual assessment was not routinely conducted with these children. Nevertheless, the cognitive skills of these children were assessed for the purposes of this research. Table 5-3 sets out background information on the sample, while Table 5-4 shows the results of the assessments of cognitive skills.

Procedures

Video recordings were made of the children's communicative behaviour in the three classroom contexts. External microphones suspended from the ceiling led to a sound mixer and the video recorder. Procedures were established for transcribing the communicative behaviour from the videotapes and for training two research assistants to do this work, thus ensuring the reliability and validity of the resulting data.

Analysis of Communicative Acts

Examination of videotapes from the pilot study led to refinements of the initially postulated list of pragmatic functions appropriate to this population. Table 5-5 is an abbreviated version of the distribution of pragmatic functions generated by the research sample during the pilot study.

Transcription, Coding and Analysis of the Data

Videotaped observations were made for all children as previously discussed. After analysing the data from Context 1 observations, it

Table 5-5: Overview of pragmatic functions.

Category	Description
1. Reach/take*	• objects held by another person
2. Affiliate	• seek out another person, usually an adult • seek physical contact: take hand, lean on person for comfort
3. Request	• objects (includes taking, as gestural request) • for action, permission • for information • for clarification (some repetitions)
4. Answer	• give information or yes/no responses to the questions of others • comply, or attempt to comply, with another's request • refuse to comply, or disagree with another • repeat words or actions of another • acknowledge another's communicative act
5. Describe (unsolicited)	• point to, show objects or events • label objects (includes counting) • give information about the context or events
6. Interact	• approach, give objects, catch another's attention • social greeting, conversation boundary marker • reject the approach of another • protest (complain about listener behaviour or other context event) • admonish, control or correct the behaviour of another • threaten, by word or action • joke, play, express pleasure to another • tease, defy
7. Non-communicative or unclear intent	• uninterpretable utterance or behaviour, unclear communicative function

*Included as separate categories in the study, following pilot study.

was decided to conduct subsequent analyses with contrasting subsets of the sample. These were to include (1) the four most frequent communicators; and (2) the four children who made fewest communicative attempts. The eight children were identified for the complete analysis in the following manner. From Context 1 observations, it was possible to identify, in each of the two classes, the two children who were most communicative and the two children who were least communicative. In this way, eight children were identified for the data analysis for all three contexts. This procedure provided the opportunity to compare features of the communicative behaviour of high-rate and low-rate communicating children across three contexts.

A procedure was developed for the transcription of the communicative behaviour of the research sample from the video recordings. An 80-column layout sheet was adapted for manual transcription by observers of a range of features of the children's communicative behaviour, including semantic, syntactic, phonological as well as pragmatic elements (Linfoot, 1987). Of concern to this study were the data on the pragmatic functions of communicative acts, using the list presented in Table 5-5. A training manual and videotape were prepared for training observers in the transcription and coding processes and for establishing their reliability.

Validation Procedures for the Transcription of Video-recorded Data

A first step in ensuring the integrity of the transcribed data was to adapt the procedure known as "triangulation" from the accounts offered by Adelman (1981) and Bernstein and Tiegerman (1989). Adelman described the procedure as getting people whose actions or communicative behaviours have been observed to give an account of those actions after a record (such as an audiotape or videotape) of those actions has been replayed for them (p 79). Commenting on the use of this technique, Brinker and Goldbart (1981, p 39) noted that when mothers adventitiously offered interpretations of their children's utterances, it was clear that more complex linguistic forms were involved than were apparent to the observers.

In the present study, the subjects being observed lacked the communication skills to report on their own communicative behaviour from videotapes. However, an adaptation of the process was used, in which each of the two class teachers was asked to report on the communicative acts of a number of children in their own class. This process was accomplished by getting the teachers to view the videotape for each observation, to watch the target child's communicative behaviour and then to record on audiotape their own interpretation of each of that child's communicative acts. The researcher later made transcripts of the teachers' accounts and compared these with the communicative acts being transcribed from the video recordings of the children.

Table 5-6 shows the results of comparing the transcripts of the teachers' and the research observer's accounts of the communicative behaviour of the four children in each class who were included in the final sample. The observations compared in this table were collected from Context 1 on the first occasion. A percentage agreement index is used to show the proportion of communicative acts identified and interpreted by the teacher that were identified and interpreted in the same way by the research observer.

Table 5-6 indicates that generally high levels of agreement were achieved between the children's teachers and the research observer in identifying the presence of communicative behaviour with respect to both the detail of the words spoken and the other actions considered to be communicative. The two cases of low agreement levels (50%) were for children producing very few communicative behaviours in those observation sessions, indicating the need for adequate numbers of observations in order to obtain useful data. This adaptation of the triangulation procedure appears to have been a useful strategy in attesting to at least the validity of these observers' transcripts.

Reliability Procedures for the Transcription of Video-recorded Data

Table 5-7 shows reliability estimates for the occurrence of communicative acts and Table 5-8 for the assignment of pragmatic functions to those acts. Some rather interesting information is revealed by these tables. In this study, it appears that more difficulty was experienced in having the two observers independently reach the same judgement as to whether a child's particular behaviour should be judged to be communicative. For those actions of children that

Table 5-6: Agreement between class teachers and research observer on occurrence of children's communicative acts.

Child	Acts agreed	Acts not agreed	Extra acts reported by teacher	Per cent agreement
01	11	3	2	68
02	2	0	2	50
07	38	0	6	86
08	61	13	3	79
09	11	0	11	50
10	34	4	4	81
15	80	10	6	83
16	70	10	8	79

were so judged, Table 5-8 suggests that observers were able to reach "reasonable" agreement in interpreting communicative intent, or pragmatic function.

Indeed, this finding echoes the observation, also noted by Brinker and Goldbart (1981), that greatest difficulty was obtained in getting observers to agree upon the transcript. In the present study, observer-differences in the identification of communicative behaviour were often able to be accounted for in ways that were not at odds with the aims of the research. For example, a child said the word "no" and shook his head from side to side a few seconds later, in one observation sample. One of the transcribers interpreted this as one communicative act, while the other felt that the short delay between the two behaviours warranted the interpretation that two communicative acts were intended. The observers agreed in this instance as to the communicative intent of the actions. Certainly, as Table 5-8 indicates, the assignment of communicative intent was able to be achieved at reasonably high levels of interobserver agreement.

Results

The stability of Context 1 data was observed by comparing the distribution of functions from the first half of observation sessions with those from the second-half data. In addition, comparisons of function

Table 5-7: Inter-observer reliability estimates for the occurrence of communicative acts.

	Context 1	Context 2	Context 3
Acts agreed on by observers KL and IR	38	36	10
Additional acts reported by KL	12	18	6
Additional acts reported by IR	9	10	3
Total no. of acts in this sample	59	64	19
Percent agreement on occurrence of communicative acts	64.4	56.25	52.6

Table 5-8: Inter-observer agreement on the coding of pragmatic functions.

	Context 1	Context 2	Context 3
Agreements on coding	28	28	8
Disagreements on coding	10	8	2
No. of acts in this sample	38	36	10
Percent coding agreement	73.6	77.7	80

distributions were made over repeated observation sessions for each context setting.

Effects due to teaching context and to ability level were examined in tabulated data. Planned contrast analyses of these data were also made using a repeated measures analysis of variance on selected linguistic variates. An account of these procedures may be found in Huck, Cormier and Bounds (1974) or at a more detailed level in Lindman (1974). These showed the effects due to teaching context, to ability level within the sample and to interaction effects.

Pragmatic Functions in Context 1 Sessions

Table 5-9 presents a histogram summary of the communicative functions demonstrated by the whole sample in Context 1 lessons. Much of the communicative behaviour shown by children in Context 1 was involved with complying with teacher or other requests.

Pragmatic Functions and Discourse Role

The data on pragmatic functions shown in Table 5-9 are more interesting when viewed in relation to the discourse or conversational role of the communicative behaviour in which they occur. Table 5-10 illustrates the pragmatic functions of the sample in morning talk sessions, divided according to initiation and response conversational roles.

The data presented in Table 5-10 are illustrated in Figure 5-1. Here, the interaction between discourse roles and the pragmatic functions of the children's communicative behaviour in Context 1 can be seen more clearly.

Figure 5-1 indicates that most of the communicative behaviour of the sample in this context was made up of responding discourse roles. However, 42% of all of this communicative behaviour was concerned with complying with the teacher's requests, either verbally

Table 5-9: Pragmatic functions of the total sample for Context 1.

Category description	Frequency	Proportions of sample
Take/reach for object held by another	25	.04
Affiliate	82	.15
Request	37	.07
Comply/answer	245	.43
Describe (unasked)	42	.07
Interact	82	.15
Uninterpretable/function unclear	53	.09
Total	566	1.0

Table 5-10: Pragmatic functions in relation to discourse roles for communicative acts in Context 1.

Discourse roles	Functions								
	Reach	Affiliate	Request	Comply	Describe	Interact	Unclear	Total	Proportion
Initiation									
Proportion	(.03)	(.11)	(.04)	(.01)	(.05)	(.06)	(.04)		(.34)
Number	18	62	22	6	30	35	20	193	
Response									
Proportion	(.01)	(.04)	(.03)	(.42)	(.02)	(.08)	(.06)		(.66)
Number	7	22	15	239	12	47	33	373	
Total									
Proportion	(.04)	(.15)	(.07)	(.43)	(.07)	(.14)	(.10)		(1.0)
Number	25	84	37	245	42	82	53	566	

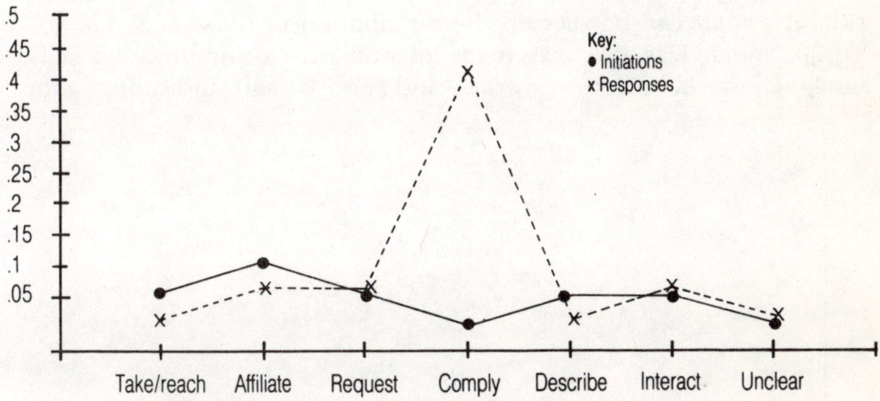

Figure 5-1: Interaction between pragmatic functions and discourse roles in Context 1.

by giving information, by acknowledging the teacher's comment in some way, or by non-verbally performing some action or movement in response to the teacher's direction. Later it will be seen that, for child-initiated communications across the sample, affiliative behaviours (seeking physical contact or comfort from being held or cuddled by the teacher) were most often observed in Context 1.

Pragmatic Functions by Developmental Level

The 16 children of whom observations were made in the initial taping of Context 1 were arranged in two developmental age levels. The first group consisted of children scoring below six months on the Bayley Scales of Infant Development (Bayley, 1969); children in the second group all scored above 23–30 months, the ceiling for the Bayley Scales. This allowed the observation of the effects of developmental levels (abilities) on pragmatic functions.

Figure 5-2 illustrates the pragmatic functions observed in Context 1 language lessons for the full sample and organised according to the children's developmental levels. This figure indicates some difference in the pragmatic functions used by children from the two developmental-level groupings.

For less able children (Level I), communication appears to have been mainly directed toward affiliative behaviours such as seeking physical comfort or contact usually with the teacher or teacher's aide (44% of communicative acts). Answering or complying with teachers' requests accounted for 23% of this group's communication and was the next-largest category.

For the more able group (Level II), Figure 5-2 indicates that a much larger number of communicative acts occurred. However, a considerable shift can be seen in the distribution of those acts. For this group, much less use was made of affiliative communicative acts, while those behaviours (verbal and non-verbal) indicating com-

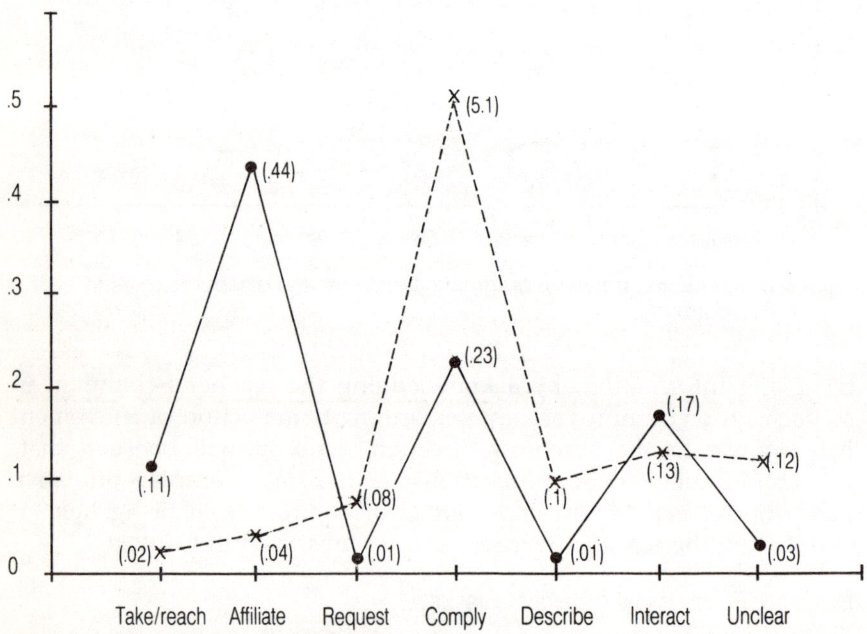

Figure 5-2: Interaction between pragmatic functions and developmental levels of subjects in Context 1.

Code: • Level I subjects (N = 8), developmental ages <6 months
× Level II subjects (N = 8), developmental ages >23 months (Bayley, 1969)

pliance with teacher requests showed a considerable increase. This change will be explored further in subsequent analyses of the data.

Within-session Stability

The following analysis compares the frequencies of pragmatic functions observed for each individual when the observation session for each was divided into two equal time intervals. Table 5-11 shows that very similar patterns are evident across the two halves. The exception concerns taking/reaching for objects from another person, where apparently greater use of communication for that purpose was observed in the second half. Nevertheless, the proportional distribution of pragmatic functions across the two observation periods does appear to be generally consistent.

Between-session Stability for Context 1

This analysis was planned to investigate the stability of pragmatic functions recorded across repeated observations of Context 1 conditions. Eight children's data were used in this and subsequent analyses, utilising the procedures and for the reasons discussed earlier.

Context 1 repetitions occurred at approximately 8 weeks (first repetition) and 16 weeks (second repetition) from the initial observation session. For each observation session, group use of pragmatic functions is reported as proportions and as frequency data in Table 5-12. It is interesting to observe that these combined data show that observed functions of communication were almost identical for the different recording sessions in this context.

Table 5-12 shows a very consistent pattern for pragmatic functions of communicative behaviours on repeated observations in Context 1. This pattern is most evident when looking at the combined subjects'

Table 5-11: Stability of pragmatic functions in observation sessions of Context 1, showing proportions (and frequencies) of communicative acts for grouped data.

Time*	Pragmatic functions							
	Take/reach	Affiliate	Request	Comply	Describe	Interact	Unclear	Total
1st half	.004 (2)	.081 (46)	.041 (23)	.226 (128)	.051 (29)	.076 (43)	.06 (34)	.538 (305)
2nd half	.041 (23)	.063 (36)	.025 (14)	.208 (118)	.021 (12)	.071 (40)	.034 (19)	.462 (262)
Totals	.044 (25)	.145 (82)	.065 (37)	.434 (246)	.072 (41)	.146 (83)	.093 (53)	1.0 (567)

*Actual observation times varied slightly for different children because of variations in classroom routines. All children's observation sessions were divided into two equal durations for this analysis.

Table 5-12: Stability of pragmatic functions over repeated observations in Context 1 for eight subjects (grouped).

Observation	Take/reach	Affiliate	Request	Comply	Describe	Interact	Unclear	Total (rounded)	Rate/minute
1	.03 (11)	.13 (44)	.04 (14)	.49 (170)	.07 (25)	.18 (61)	.06 (22)	1.0 (347)	1.96
2	.006 (3)	.14 (70)	.04 (20)	.54 (265)	.06 (31)	.17 (83)	.04 (21)	1.0 (493)	2.2
3	.003 (1)	.16 (62)	.01 (4)	.54 (211)	.08 (30)	.17 (65)	.09 (36)	1.0 (409)	2.22

Table 5-13: Stability of pragmatic functions over repeated observations in Context 2 for eight subjects (grouped).

Observation	Take/reach	Affiliate	Request	Comply	Describe	Interact	Unclear	Total (rounded)	Rate/minute
1	.04 (11)	.06 (16)	.12 (33)	.52 (143)	.11 (30)	.10 (29)	.05 (14)	1.0 (276)	1.82
2	.01 (3)	.05 (13)	.15 (37)	.42 (104)	.04 (13)	.22 (56)	.1 (24)	1.0 (250)	1.60
3	.04 (8)	.13 (29)	.16 (34)	.42 (93)	.05 (11)	.12 (27)	.08 (18)	1.0 (220)	1.56

data. However, it was also confirmed when comparing each individual's data from repeated observations in Context 1. These data may suggest that at least Context 1 classroom conditions have a powerful and consistent influence over the pragmatic purposes for which these children used their communicative behaviour.

Stability in Other Teaching Contexts

Context 2 stability data are presented in Table 5-13. Here, proportional stability in the pragmatic functions of communicative behaviour across widely spaced observation sessions of Context 2 conditions appears to be quite high.

Stability of pragmatic functions observed under Context 3 conditions was analysed in the same way, but only two observation sessions were recorded in Context 3. Routine in the school prevented the setting up of Context 3 conditions for what would have been the second repetition. Table 5-14 presents the stability data for Context 3 in grouped-subject form.

These grouped data also suggest stability between the two observation sessions in Context 3 conditions. There is a decrease in proportional use from .44 to .23 for the answer/comply function, which is the largest difference reported in Table 5-14. Nevertheless,

Table 5-14: Stability of pragmatic functions across repeated observations in Context 3 for eight subjects (grouped).

Observation	Take/reach	Affiliate	Request	Comply	Describe	Interact	Unclear	Total (rounded)	Rate/minute
1	.03	.05	.12	.44	.05	.26	.05	1.0	
	(7)	(11)	(28)	(98)	(11)	(58)	(12)	(225)	1.86
2	.04	.13	.14	.23	.07	.33	.07	1.0	
	(10)	(30)	(32)	(55)	(16)	(78)	(16)	(237)	1.51

Table 5-15: Pragmatic functions in three classroom contexts for eight children.

Context	Pragmatic function							
	Take/reach	Affiliate	Request	Comply	Describe	Interact	Unclear	Total
1	.02	.14	.02	.52	.07	.17	.06	1.0
2	.02	.08	.14	.46	.07	.15	.08	1.0
3	.03	.09	.13	.34	.06	.28	.07	1.0

the pattern of pragmatic functions observed in the two observations in Context 3 conditions remains generally consistent.

To summarise the discussion so far, it is argued that this methodology has produced data on children's communicative functions that have been demonstrated to be stable both within and between observation sessions involving similar teaching contexts. It has also demonstrated that stable patterns of data were obtained for each of the three teaching contexts investigated.

Concerning the data collected in Context 1, it was found that by far the greatest use to which children's communicative behaviour was put concerned complying with teacher requests, by either vocal or other methods. Further analysis showed that pattern to be related to children's cognitive developmental level, with less able children complying less and engaging in more affiliative behaviour involving clinging to the teacher and holding the teacher's hand when possible.

Effects of Context Variation on Pragmatic Functions

An overall view of possible context effects was obtained by presenting data on the use of communicative functions in different contexts as proportions (Table 5-15).

These data suggest the possibility of change in the use of a number of pragmatic functions in different communicative contexts. To assist the visual examination of these trends, the Table 5-15 data are presented in Figure 5-3.

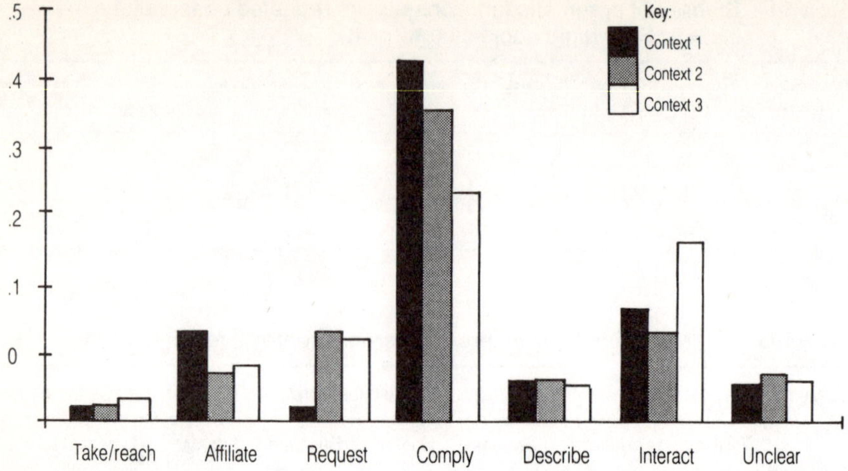

Figure 5-3: Pragmatic functions in three classroom contexts for eight children.

This presentation makes evident the effects of context on children's communicative behaviour. First, there appears to be a decrease across contexts in what has been termed affiliative behaviour, where the child clings to or reaches for the teacher or another adult for apparent physical comfort. Affiliative behaviour seems to occur most frequently in the more highly structured lessons where children are asked to attend to the teacher's directions throughout the lesson. However, this apparent trend was not significant at the 5% level in the planned contrast analyses performed on the data (see Table 5-17 below).

Children's requesting behaviours, which are more likely to be child-initiated acts than, say, answering behaviours, appear to occur more frequently in Contexts 2 and 3, where less teacher structuring of the environment occurs. This result is suggested by the data shown in Table 5-15 and Figure 5-3. However, Table 5-16 shows that this effect occurred only among the more able children within the sample. These were the children more likely to request in all contexts and especially in Context 2 and 3 conditions. Nevertheless, the trend shown by these data was not sufficiently strong to achieve statistical significance (see Table 5-17).

The complying and answering communicative function did occur more frequently in Context 1, achieving statistical significance ($p < .05$) (Table 5-17). Upon close examination, it can be seen that the setting and activities of Context 1, being highly teacher-directed, are structured to elicit compliance with teacher directions, both through action and through language or other communicative behaviour from the children. Interestingly, the children's ability is also related to the act of complying and answering ($p < .01$) with an interaction between ability and context effects also established (Table 5-17).

Finally, the interactional function is of interest. Though not reaching significance at the .05 level, a strong trend toward an increase in the use of this communicative function is apparent in Context 3, where teacher-structuring of the classroom is minimised and where maximum opportunity for child-initiated interactional communicative behaviour might be expected to occur.

Contextual Effects and Developmental Level Effects on Pragmatic Functions

The influence of developmental level on the distribution of children's pragmatic functions in each observation context is examined in Table 5-16.

These data are also presented as proportions of each group's communicative acts for each function. Affiliative behaviour showed a trend toward almost exclusive use by lower-ability children, which was apparent in all lesson contexts though its use gradually decreased as lessons became less structured.

Conversely, requesting (objects or information) tended to be more likely to be used by both ability groups in the less structured lesson contexts. This trend was stronger for the higher-ability group.

As noted above, a context–ability interaction effect is present for the complying communicative function ($p < .05$), where greater use of this function was observed for the more able group. For that group, the use of complying was related to context structure.

Describing was used more frequently by the more able group ($p < .05$) but not differently across contexts. Social interactive uses of communicative behaviour appeared most often in the least-structured lesson context (Context 3) and was similar for both groups.

Table 5-16: Pragmatic functions in three classroom contexts for the sample arranged in two ability levels.

Context	Level	Pragmatic function							
		Take/reach	Affiliate	Request	Comply	Describe	Interact	Unclear	Total
1	1	.04	.45	.01	.28	0	.20	.02	1.0
	2	0	.02	.04	.62	.10	.16	.06	1.0
2	1	.08	.33	.02	.42	.02	.12	.01	1.0
	2	.02	.03	.16	.46	.08	.16	.09	1.0
3	1	.06	.29	.10	.23	0	.30	.02	1.0
	2	.03	.03	.14	.36	.08	.29	.07	1.0

Statistical Analysis

To assist in analysing the data on communicative behaviour, a series of planned contrasts was conducted using an analysis of variance (ANOVA) repeated measures design. A discussion of the use of this procedure may be found in Hays (1981), Huck, Cormier and Bounds (1974) and Lindman (1974). On the basis of earlier research with other populations, it was predicted that communicative behaviour in highly teacher-directed lessons would tend to be restricted to the answering and complying pragmatic function, and greater use of child-initiated functions involving requesting, social interaction and unsolicited describing functions would occur in less teacher-structured lessons. As a result, planned contrasts were developed to test the following effects upon a range of behaviours associated with linguistic functioning, and were organised around the model involving the *form, content* and *use* dimensions proposed by Bloom and Lahey (1978).

1. Do lower-functioning children differ from higher-functioning children?
2. Does Context 1 differ from the average of Contexts 2 and 3?
3. Does Context 2 differ from Context 3?
4. Are there interactional effects between developmental level and lesson context?

These questions were applied to selected variables involving pragmatic, semantic and discourse functions, mode of communication, intonation, eye-pointing and communicative match. Data on the ANOVA comparison are reported in detail by Linfoot (1987) and are summarised in Table 5-17. The following discussion will be limited to contextual effects on the pragmatics variables in this study.

A number of anticipated outcomes concerning children's pragmatic skills were found. It was not surprising that ability level had a significant effect on the use of a number of pragmatic functions. Its strongest influence was on the answer/comply function, where higher-ability children used this function more frequently than their developmentally younger peers. The describing, unclear and the responding discourse functions were also used more often by the more able group, who also demonstrated considerably more communicative behaviour. Nevertheless, this greater use of communication by the more able group was not represented across all communicative functions. Requests and social interactions, both more likely to be child-initiated uses of communication, were not used more frequently by any one ability group. Indeed, because of the use of affiliative behaviour by two of the lower-ability group children, there was a trend for this function to be associated with that group.

The other important area for analysis concerns the effects of the lesson context on children's use of communicative functions. The only clear results were for the comply/answer function, where Context 1 was associated significantly ($p < .05$) with this function's use (see Table 5-17). There was also an interaction effect between ability level and the planned contrast involving Context 1 for comply/answer. Context 1 was also significantly associated with the responding discourse mode, as shown in Table 5-17.

These results were not unexpected for Context 1, where the strong control of the teacher in that context meant that there was little opportunity for child-initiated interactions. Most communication involved responding to teacher directions, often by practising responses, greeting forms and the names of people and objects within the classroom. This communicative context appeared most suitable for teachers to help children master particular linguistic forms or understand semantic content, but less suitable for developing social interactive and autonomous use of communicative behaviour.

Of particular interest, therefore, should be the effects of the less-structured contexts on eliciting children's use of the more socially appropriate communicative functions. The request function appeared to be used relatively more frequently in Contexts 2 and 3. However, inspection of the individual data summaries (Linfoot, 1987) shows that a large difference in favour of Contexts 2 and 3 by one particular pupil (#8) does account for the trend suggested by the grouped data. In fact, most of the children did not request very often in *any context*, and it is this reluctance by children with intellectual disabilities to initiate communication that has been the concern of this research. Nevertheless, despite the absence of a statistically significant effect (Table 5-17), the data for individuals show that five of the eight children used somewhat more requesting behaviours in Contexts 2 and 3 than in Context 1, suggesting that those two contexts may have been more conducive to this use of communication.

For the social interaction function, the planned contrast analyses show a similar pattern of results as for requesting, with one child displaying considerably more of this behaviour than the others. Similarly, a trend for the initiation discourse function was noticed for the Context 2/3 contrast, suggesting increased use in Context 3.

An unexpected outcome of this research concerned the children's use of communicative behaviour for obtaining emotional comfort and physical contact from one of the adults present. Termed "affiliative behaviour", these actions were considered to be communicative in this research although it was not always clear whether this behaviour met all the criteria established for defining a communicative act (Linfoot, 1987). While the behaviours were clearly intentional, were directed toward an adult and appeared to give the child some comfort through the physical proximity of the adult, there was often no sense in which any linguistic meaning or symbolic content could be associated with the act. Table 5-17 indicates observed trends for greater use of affiliative behaviour by lower-functioning children than by more able children, and for this behaviour to be more evident in the structured setting of Context 1 than in the less-structured settings.

Examination of the analyses suggests that contextual effects upon the various linguistic measures may not have been as powerful as predicted. Closer study of the original raw data shows that individual differences were often very strong. However, while strong trends existed in the predicted directions for some of the linguistic elements shown in Table 5-17, individual variability in this small sample, in-

Table 5-17: Summary of ability and context effects on the communicative behaviour of the sample, showing F tests and significant levels (Hays, 1981).

Element	Ability effects	Context effects	Ability–context interaction
Form			
verbal	trend G2 > G1 (F = 5.082)	trend 2C1 > C2 + C3 (F = 5.408)	trend 2C1 > C2 + C3 (F = 5.160)
mean length of utterance	G2 > G1a		
uninterpretable vocalisation	G2 > G1a		
intonation fall	G2 > G1a	2C1 > C2 + C3a	
intonation unclear		C3 > C2a	
avert eyes		2C1 > C2 + C3a	
Content			
performative	G2 > G1a	C2 > C3a	
naming	G2 > G1a	2C1 > C2 + C3a	2C1 > C2 + C3a
desired object		C2 + C3 > 2C1a	C2 + C3 > 2C1a
agent	G2 > G1a	2C1 > C2 + C3b	2C1 > C2 + C3b
full match spk	G2 > G1b		
part match spk	G2 > G1a	2C1 > C2 + C3a	
Use			
affiliate	trend G1 > G2	trend 2C1 > C2 + C3	trend 2C1 > C2 + C3
request		trend C2 + C3 > 2C1	
comply	G2 > G1b	2C1 > C2 + C3a	2C1 > C2 + C3a
describe	G2 > G1a		
interact		trend C3 > C2 (F = 5.777)	
unclear	G2 > G1a		
discourse initiations		trend C3 > C2 (F = 4.884)	
discourse responses	G2 > G1b	2C1 > C2 + C3a	

Code: G = Ability group; C = Context
Levels of statistical significance a. $p < .05$; b. $p < .01$
full match spk = full match with speaker's meaning;
part match spk = partial match with speaker's meaning.

cluding cases of zero entries for some children on most elements, resulted in a number of trends not reaching statistical significance at the .05 level.

To summarise the findings so far, it is suggested, nevertheless, that Context 1 conditions appeared to be associated with complying and answering functions of communication and possibly with affiliative behaviour for the developmentally youngest children in the sample. Clear evidence was not found for increased use of any particular functions in Contexts 2 and 3, although there appeared to be a trend for interactional and discourse initiation functions to be used more often in Context 3 than 2. For a small number of children, the request function appears to have been used in Contexts 2 and 3 more often than in Context 1.

The difficulties of identifying group trends in these analyses are illustrated by the following case study discussion, where attention is drawn to the idiosyncratic nature of one child's communicative behaviour.

Sample Case Study Analysis

In the following analysis, an account is offered of the communicative behaviour of one of the children in the sample. The account also includes relevant information on the child's physical development and available medical information. Communicative behaviour is described where appropriate, in terms of its phonological, semantic, syntactic and pragmatic features. Finally, some discussion centres on the bizarre and non-communicative vocal behaviours demonstrated, with a view to speculating about their possible communicative intent along the lines suggested by Barnett (1986) and by Wetherby and Prutting (1984).

Subject #2, R.

This 11-year-old boy produced the smallest amount of communicative behaviour observed in the research sample. Institutionalised over a long period, R. suffered the effects of a variety of developmental disabilities. At birth, which was induced after a 43-week pregnancy, R.'s difficulties included metabolic disorders of digestion, neonatal jaundice and profound epileptic seizures, while a vision problem became apparent in the weeks following. His parents were described in the hospital records as "young and immature, with a history of mental retardation".

During the observation period of the present research, R.'s epileptic condition was controlled by medication. His physical appearance was that of a child younger than his 11 years, but with no characteristic appearance suggesting retardation. In all observation sessions, he spent a lot of time flapping his hands, clapping in a ritualistic fashion, or fixing the researcher or other adults in the room with long, relentless stares or smiles which conveyed little in the way of clear communicative intent.

R. was unable to produce recognisable vocalisations, but during many observation sessions he emitted very low moaning sounds which appeared to serve as accompaniment to his ritualistic hand-flapping and clapping. Occasionally he produced a scream, possibly in imitation of another child in the class who screamed quite frequently. However, he did sometimes use a smile or laugh apparently meaningfully, as a response to the teacher when, for example, she praised him for an earlier response.

Research data show that R. used a narrow range of communicative functions, being restricted largely to affiliative behaviours and complying with teacher requests. An interesting exception concerns requesting. It was only in one Context 2 session that an example of this communicative function was used by R. In that session, a nurse had been giving him a drink as part of the "morning tea" ritual and had just removed the cup as he was swallowing his juice. When finished, R. clapped his hands vigorously, rather in the stereotyped manner frequently observed in these sessions, and stared fixedly at the cup of juice. The nurse interpreted the clapping-and-staring sequence as an indication that he wanted more juice. He certainly accepted the offer of more juice most enthusiastically and, after drinking some, repeated the sequence of clapping and staring at the cup.

This sequence is of interest for a number of reasons. In the first place, it illustrates the way in which the child's rather ambiguous behaviours were interpreted by the nurse as communicative, in the absence of a clear expression of intent. The lack of a vocal request, even the lack of eye-pointing between the desired object (juice) and the nurse, who was the only possible instrument for satisfying this need, made R.'s behaviour appear to be a very primitive form of request. At best, his behaviour seemed to indicate the object he desired, but he did not address his request to another person. The nurse's interpretation of his actions as a request illustrated the process described by Lock (1980), in which meanings that are attributed to the actions of infants reinforce those actions which are thereafter performed by infants with intent.

The second interesting aspect of this sequence is the context in which it occurred. Being less teacher-directed than Context 1, this session included activities relating to basic physiological needs (food and drink) and was not really part of a formal language lesson. Thus, the incidental interactions prompted by a physical need provided the most useful context for this particular child in these observation sequences to demonstrate what may have been a form of requesting behaviour. That context, together with the presence of an adult who was able to recognise that primitive request form and interpret it for R., could have important implications for the education processes employed with such individuals. For children as developmentally disabled as R., one might now expect that most opportunities for the development of communication skills might occur within the context of physical care-giving in one-to-one situations. For the present research, these findings illustrate the appropriateness of Context 2 conditions for observing primitive requesting behaviours. They also show, however, that the frequency of such occurrences is very low and is therefore unlikely to contribute to a statistically significant comparison of contexts when the grouped data are considered.

Observations of this youngster's interactions have provided very limited evidence for the expression of communicative intent by R. His primitive form of requesting behaviour could be seen as the beginnings of the development of communicative intent. This behaviour was not generalised to other settings, however, and there was no evidence for his use of the requesting function for other objects or actions. What may be important, however, is that the intentional behaviour did occur in Context 2 observation conditions.

Summary and Discussion

Verbal and non-verbal communicative behaviour of institutionalised children with severe intellectual disability was analysed in relation to pragmatic functions using over 20 hours of videotaped observations in three lesson contexts. Stable and consistent use of a pragmatics-coding taxonomy was demonstrated, although some difficulty was found in this study, as with others, in establishing observer agreement on the occurrence of communicative behaviour.

Some differences in pragmatic functions of communication were noted between two groups of subjects with different developmental levels. Differences were also noted in the use of certain pragmatic functions and interpersonal interactions when teachers arranged the lesson context so that they had varying degrees of control over classroom activity, although contextual effects were not as strong as predicted.

Nevertheless, the observed contextual effects may be important in dealing with the often-reported inappropriate usage of communication by people with intellectual disability, often after participation in various forms of "language" training (McLean & Snyder-McLean, 1978; Bedrosian & Prutting, 1978; Leudar, 1981). The present study has suggested that the ways in which the classroom context (in school settings) is arranged may have some influence on the distribution of children's communicative functions. The unwillingness of many institutionalised individuals to use, or to use more appropriately, the language skills they possess may be changed by an increased use of care environments that emphasise a minimum of teacher control over activities and communication. Instead, greater use may be made of social-interactive settings where interpersonal interaction becomes an outcome of a shared activity of group members. Participation in turn-taking and socialisation games have been recommended to this end (Conant, Budoff, Hecht & Morse, 1984; Edmonson & Han, 1983; Jeffre & Cheseldine, 1984; Linfoot, 1983).

Procedures such as those employed in this study appear to hold some value for practitioners in identifying the pragmatic characteristics of their clients' communication skills. This should lead to the identification, in particular individuals or groups, of the pragmatic functions that need to be incorporated in the communicative behaviour. The effect of particular classroom contexts on the use of pragmatic functions of communication as shown in the study can be considered when planning communication intervention programs.

References

Adelman, C. (1981). *Uttering, muttering*. London: Grant McIntyre Ltd.

Barnett, J. (1986). *Communication with persons who have language handicaps: A transactional perspective*. Paper presented to the AGSOMD Conference, Sydney.

Bates, E. (1976). *Language and context: The acquisition of pragmatics*. New York: Academic Press.

Bates, E., Benigni, L., Bretherton, I., Camaioni, L. & Volterra, V. (1977). From gesture to the first word: On cognitive and social prerequisites. In M. Lewis & L.A. Rosenblum (eds), *Interaction, conversation and the development of language*. New York: John Wiley & Sons.

Bayley, N. (1969). Bayley scales of infant development. NY: Psychological Corporation.

Bedrosian, J.L. & Prutting, C.A. (1978). Communicative performance of mentally retarded adults in four conversational settings. *Journal of Speech and Hearing Research 21*, 79–95

Bernstein, D.K. & Tiegerman, E. (1989). *Language and communication disorders in children* (2nd edn). Columbus: Charles E. Merrill.

Bloom, L. & Lahey, M. (1978). *Language development and language disorders*. New York: John Wiley & Sons.

Bloomfield, L. (1933). *Language*. New York: Holt, Rinehart & Winston.

Brinker, R.P. & Goldbart, J. (1981). The problem of reliability in the study of early communication skills. *British Journal of Psychology 72*, 27–41.

Brown, R. (1973). *A first language: The early stages*. Cambridge, Mass.: Harvard University Press.

Calculator, S. & Dollaghen, C. (1982). The use of communication boards in a residential setting: An evaluation. *Journal of Speech and Hearing Disorders 47*, 281–87.

Cardosa-Martins, C., Mervis, C.B. & Mervis, C.A. (1985). Early vocabulary acquisition by children with Down syndrome. *American Journal of Mental Deficiency 90* (2), 177–84.

Chapman, R.S. (1981). Exploring children's communicative intents. In J.F. Miller (ed.), *Assessing language production in children*. London: Edward Arnold.

Chomsky, N. (1957). *Syntactic structures*. The Hague: Mouton.

Cirrin, F.M. & Rowland, C.M. (1985). Communicative assessment of nonverbal youths with severe/profound mental retardation. *Mental Retardation 23* (2), 52–62.

Coggins, T.E. & Carpenter, R.L. (1980). The communicative intention inventory: A system for observing and coding children's early intentional communication. *Applied Psycholinguistics 2* (3), 235–51.

Conant, S., Budoff, M., Hecht, B. & Morse, R. (1984). Language intervention: A pragmatic approach. *Journal of Autism & Developmental Disorders 14* (3), 301–17.

Dore, J. (1973). *The development of speech acts*. PhD dissertation. Reproduced by University Microfilms International, London, 1978.

Dore, J. (1974). A pragmatic description of early language development. *Journal of Psycholinguistic Research 3* (4), 343–50.

Edmonson, B. & Han, S.S. (1983). Effects of socialization games on proximity and prosocial behavior of aggressive mentally retarded institutionalized women. *American Journal of Mental Deficiency 87* (4), 435–40.

Fraser, W. (1981). Clinical presentations of retarded language. In W. Fraser & R. Grieve (eds), *Communicating with normal and retarded children*. Bristol: John Wright & Sons.

Grossman, H. (1983). *Classification in mental retardation*. Washington: American Association on Mental Deficiency.

Halliday, M.A.K. (1975). *Learning how to mean: Explorations in the development of language*. London: Arnold.

Harris, J. (1984). Encouraging linguistic interactions between severely mentally handicapped children and teachers in special schools. *Special Education: Forward Trends. Research Supplement 11* (2), 17–24.

Hart, B. & Risley, T.R. (1968). Establishing use of descriptive adjectives in the spontaneous speech of disadvantaged preschool children. *Journal of Applied Behavior Analysis 1* (2) 109–20.

Hart, B. & Rogers-Warren, A. (1978). A milieu approach to teaching language. In R.L. Schiefelbusch (ed.), *Language intervention strategies*. Baltimore: University Park Press.

Hays, W.L. (1981). *Statistics* (3rd edn). NY: Holt, Rinehart & Winston.

Huck, S.W., Cormier, W.H. & Bounds, W.G. (1974). *Reading statistics and research*. NY: Harper & Row.

Jeffre, D.M. & Cheseldine, S.E. (1984). Programmed leisure intervention and the interaction patterns of severely mentally retarded adolescents: A pilot study. *American Journal of Mental Deficiency 88* (6), 619–24.

Leudar, I. (1981). Strategic communication in mental retardation. In W. Fraser & R. Grieve (eds), *Communicating with normal and retarded children*. Bristol: John Wright & Sons.

Light, J., Collier, B. & Parnes, P. (1985). Communicative interaction between young non-speaking physically disabled children and their primary caregivers (Part II: Communicative function). *Journal of Augmentative and Alternative Communication 1*, 98–106.

Lindman, H.R. (1974). *Analysing of variance in complex experimental designs*. San Francisco: W.H. Freeman.

Linfoot, K.W. (1983). Language use of mentally handicapped school children: Developing communication skills. *The ASET Journal 17*, 27–30.

Linfoot, K.W. (1987). *An investigation of communicative behaviour in institutionalised children with severe developmental delay*. PhD thesis. Sydney: Macquarie University.

Lock, A. (1980). *The guided reinvention of language*. London: Academic Press.

McCormick, L. & Schiefelbusch R.L. (1990). *Early language: An introduction* (2nd edn). Columbus: Charles E. Merrill.

McLean, J.E., McLean, L.K.S., Brady, N.C. & Etter, R. (1991). Communication profiles of two types of gestures using nonverbal persons with severe to profound mental retardation. *Journal of Speech and Hearing Research 34*, 294–308.

McLean, J.E. & Snyder-McLean, L.J. (1978). *A transactional approach to early language training*. Columbus: Charles E. Merrill.

Miller, J.F. (1981). *Assessing language production in children: Experimental procedures*. London: Edward Arnold.

Miller, J.F. (in press). Language and communication characteristics of children with Down syndrome. In A. Crocker, S. Paschel, J. Rynders & C. Tinghey (eds), *Down Syndrome: State of the art*. Baltimore: Brooks Publishing Co.

Moerk, E.L. (1977). *Pragmatic and semantic aspects of early language development*. Baltimore: University Park Press.

Nihira, K., Foster, R., Shellhaas, M. & Leland, H. (1974). *AAMD Adaptive Behavior Scale Manual*. Washington: American Association on Mental Deficiency.

O'Connor, N. & Hermelin, B. (1962). *Speech and thought in severe subnormality: An experimental study*. Oxford: Pergamon Press.

Owens, R.E. & MacDonald, J.D. (1982). Communicative uses of the early speech of non-delayed and Down syndrome children. *American Journal of Mental Deficiency 86* (5), 803–10.

Owings, N.O., McManus, M.D. & Scherer, N. (1981). A deinstitutionalized retarded adult's use of communication functions in a natural setting. *British Journal of Disorders of Communication 16* (2), 119–28.

Roth, F.P. & Spekman, N.J. (1984). Assessing the pragmatic abilities of children (Part I: Organizational framework and assessment parameters). *Journal of Speech and Hearing Disorders 49*, 2–11.

Rowland, C. (1990). Communication in the classroom for children with dual sensory impairments: Studies of teacher and child behavior. *AAC Augmentative and Alternative Communication 6*, 262–74.

Searle, J. (1969). *Speech acts*. Cambridge: Cambridge University Press.

Skinner. B.F. (1957). *Verbal behavior*. New York: Appleton-Century-Crofts.

Staats, A.W. (1968). *Language, learning and cognition*. New York: Holt, Rinehart & Winston.

Wepman, J. (1959). Auditory discrimination, speech and hearing. *Elementary School Journal 60*, 325–33.

Wetherby, A.M. & Prutting, C.A. (1984). Profiles of communicative and cognitive-social abilities in autistic children. *Journal of Speech and Hearing Research 27*, 364–77.

Chapter 6

The Use of a Synthetic Speech Output Communication Aid by a Youth with Severe Developmental Disability

Sue Healy
Cranleigh Special School
Canberra, ACT

Communication is the primary function of language (Muma, 1978) and can be seen as the process by which people initiate, develop and maintain cooperative interactions with others. Communication enhances the individual's ability to become a functional member of society, living and interacting with others in daily domestic, educational, work and recreational environments. Halliday (1975) described normal communicative functions as using language to satisfy needs (instrumental function), to exert control over the behaviour of others (regulatory function) and to share information with a communicative partner (informative function). Austin (1962) described three speech actions: perlocutions, which are acts that produce an effect on a receiver (regulatory); illocutions, which are acts that express a communicative intent of the sender (informative); and locutions, which are specific linguistic propositions used to express the sender's intent (instrumental).

Referential and pragmatic functions of communicative acts have been described by McLean and Snyder-McLean (1987). Traditional language models had tended to stress the referential function, which is the relationship between an utterance and its real world referent. More recent studies of pragmatic features of language development (Bates et al, 1975; Bates, 1976; Rees, 1978; Duchan, 1984) have led to a broader perspective on sociocommunicative functions. The pragmatic view of language sees it not only in terms of linguistic form and referential function, but also as acts carried out by a sender on a receiver.

The most effective and immediate means of communication is through the spoken word, which is the optimal and most flexible means by which communication acts can be contextually displayed. However, individuals having severe multiple disabilities are frequently unable to use functional vocal speech as a mode of communication for expressing needs, feelings and desires and for engaging in general conversational interactions. This presents major problems for those persons capable of receiving and processing language. Communication involves more than passive reception of what is being expressed by others. It is a dynamic interpersonal process in which there is a constant shifting of the roles of expresser and sender (Schiefelbusch, 1980).

Many disabled persons indicate an ability to express themselves in some form, using, for example, body movement, finger- and/or eye-pointing and facial expression. Some of these people have been able to augment communication and supplement and/or facilitate vocal communication by using an alternative means of expression.

Augmentative Communication Systems

Augmentative communication systems can be placed into two major categories, unaided and aided (Lloyd, 1985). *Unaided systems* can best be described as those necessitating body movements that may be termed dynamic, such as signing systems, sign language and pantomime (Musselwhite & St Louis, 1988). These systems do not require equipment or devices. The use of unaided techniques depends largely on the situational context, communication partners, and the physical and cognitive abilities of the user. The use of natural gestures restricts the vocabularly available to express an idea, and manual signing can only be understood by others who are familiar with the rules and gestures of the signing system used (Nietupski & Hamre-Nietupski, 1979).

Interest in communication processes such as pragmatics and non-vocal behaviour and the trend away from the preoccupation with sentence structure and vocabulary acquisition have been major features of the development and use of *aided communication systems* (Bloomberg & Johnson, 1991; Houghton, Bronicki & Guess, 1987; Mirenda, Iacono & Williams, 1990).

Non-electronic aids include communication boards involving the use of visual material such as photographs, line drawings, letters, words, and graphic symbol systems such as Rebus, Computer Pictographs for Communication (COMPICS) and Blissymbolics (Bernstein & Tiegerman, 1989). The selection of a symbol system depends on the user's physical and cognitive skills and those of significant communicative partners. Users will not be able to effect successful communicative interactions with others if they cannot understand what a symbol represents. The more iconic the symbols are, in that they are more pictorially representative of the referents, the easier they are to learn (Clarke, 1981). The communication board is usually portable, easy to make and can be adapted to meet the physical range of movement of the user. Positioning of the board to enable easy access must be considered, allowing the user to indicate the desired message through finger-pointing, eye-pointing, head gesture or with the use of a head pointer.

COMPICS, developed in a joint venture by the Swinburne Institute of Technology in Victoria and the Victorian Symbol Standardisation Committee, are iconic symbols suitable for the communicative needs of people with moderate to severe developmental disability. Special schools in Canberra have found COMPICS to be most effective in communication programs for these students from primary (elementary school) through to secondary (high school) level. Blissymbolics (Bernstein & Tiegerman, 1989), on the other hand, are less iconic and are appropriate for those with higher levels of cognitive functioning. In this system, symbols, pictures, words and drawings may be used in a combination that suits the abilities and needs of the user.

Advances in technology have made it possible to augment communication through the use of electronic aids, which have opened up a wide range of possibilities for non-vocal persons (Vanderheiden, 1982). These devices can assist non-vocal persons to be more effective in communication, giving them opportunities to express themselves through electronically controlled visual and/or auditory systems, instead of being placed in passive receiver roles or being frustrated in their efforts to communicate with others who do not understand symbol systems.

Electronic aids produce visual displays, printouts, prerecorded speech and synthesised speech which can be programmed to user needs. The choice of input systems, such as single or multiple switches, joysticks, keyboards and magnetised switches, depends on the user's individual range of movement, visual and auditory capabilities and ability to read and write. A wide range of electronic computer-based devices is on the market, and the range continues to expand as technological research advances.

There are two basic types of input techniques used with electronic devices: direct selection and scanning. *Direct selection* involves the user selecting the desired item by using a keyboard, eye gaze, finger-pointing or an optical head pointer. This type of input technique is not the most feasible for people with severe gross motor deficits as uncontrolled physical movements can result in inappropriate activation. For these people a scanning device would be more accessible and appropriate. *Scanning* with electronic displays involves the user activating a signal, usually with a switch, to indicate the desired item from a scanned sequence. Scanning device systems include a computer screen on which a light or cursor moves in linear fashion, scans group items or moves by direct scanning. In linear scanning, items are scanned one at a time along the line until the user indicates the desired item. This can be a time-consuming process. Group item scanning involves row-column scanning whereby the user first indicates the correct row and the row items are then presented in sequence until the user indicates the desired item. In directed scanning, the type and timing of the user's direction of movement influences item selection as in using a joystick to move the indicator right, left, up, down or diagonally, with the user activating a switch to make the selection when the indicator is over the item required. The types of output produced by electronic devices include visual output in the form of hard copy and visual display screens, which make it necessary for the user and receiver to be able to read. Auditory output forms include taped human speech and synthesised speech.

Voice output communication aids (VOCA) are becoming increasingly popular for use by non-vocal persons with severe multiple disabilities. A system now sold in many countries is the ScanWolf VOCA, which was used in the study reported below. This has a single-activator switch and is a small, portable, battery-operated device easily fixed to the tray of a wheelchair. It is a voice synthesiser with no printout or visual display screen and is available with a manual or automatic switching mode and with a linear or row-column scanning mode. This device can store up to 500 words on electronically programmable read only memory (EPROM) on each of 36 overlays. Each vocabulary overlay can accommodate 36 items which can include words and/or symbols. The voice output can relay the symbols in words.

Selecting Communication Devices to Meet User Needs

In identifying the optimal augmentative communication device for a particular user, the individual's cognitive, social, emotional and physical needs and abilities must be considered along with language abilities and communication needs. The environments in which the user moves and the potential communicative partners within these environments must be taken into account (Chapman & Miller, 1980).

The user's final communication goals must be firmly established. Musselwhite and St Louis (1988, p 18) quoted Van Tatenhove (1986) when describing the selection of a communication device:

> Rationale for selection of a primary system and a transition through systems is based on the communicative and cognitive potential of the student, his or her ability to use the system as it was intended, and the final communication goal. The question "Am I using this system simply because Johnny can learn it or because it will increase his communication and interactive potential?" must be asked.

Boltorf and De Pape (1982) suggested that, while an augmentative communication aid should be selected according to the individual user's present needs, the focus of any intervention should be based on increasing successful communicative interaction.

Effectiveness of Augmentative Communication Systems

There is some debate among researchers and authors on the use of augmentative systems as alternatives to, or substitutes for, speech (Harris & Vanderheiden, 1980). However, Musselwhite and St Louis (1988) made the following point:

> . . . if we are truly concerned about being communication oriented, as Silverman (1980) recommends, and if our primary concern is interaction as some authors suggest (Harris and Vanderheiden, 1980; Kraat, 1985), transmitting information through a non-vocal system is an acceptable function, at least initially.

Studies of the use of augmentative communication aids have found that they do not inhibit the development of speech and, perhaps more importantly, they do bring more information to the communication attempt, thus increasing intelligibility. Silverman (1980) asserted that augmentative systems improved the ability to communicate and were often accompanied by more attempts at speech. Beukelman and Yorkston (1977) concluded that the use of augmentative aids is associated with increased intelligibility. Kahn (1977) asserted that augmentative communication facilitates spontaneous attempts at verbal communication.

Augmentative communication aids have also been found to increase communicative interactions. Harris (1982) and Light, Collier and Parnes (1985) found that young children with severe to profound disabilities would use their augmentative communication aids with or without other unaided, non-vocal modes to answer questions, to request actions or objects and to clarify statements when requested to do so. However, the children tended to remain in passive respondent roles with adults controlling the interactions. The children rarely initiated communicative interaction, asked for information or made social comments. Harris stressed that communication exchanges are the responsibility of both sender and receiver and that both must have developed some skills in communicative interaction. The devices themselves cannot do the interacting.

Calculator and Bollaghen (1982) found a similar pattern of passive respondent behaviour in older children and adults with moderate to severe intellectual disabilities. Molloy (1987) found that there was no real improvement in the communicative initiations and responses of a ten-year-old subject with cerebral palsy using a Vocriss VOCA. Molloy concluded that the subject was not familiar enough with the technical operation of the Vocriss and that the size and lack of portability of the device did not offer the subject access to it at all times. Pitt (1988), in a paper presented to the seventh Australian Seminar of Technical Aid to the Disabled, reported that physically handicapped children using LightTalkers (a voice output communication aid activated by infra-red light directed by the user) tended to use the voice output mode in academic programs rather than for communication. It was found that the stored utterances, while relating to what the children wanted to communicate, did not state contextually specific messages. The listeners tended to accept the voice-synthesised message at face value. When only symbols were used, listeners tended to guess around them to understand the sender's exact message.

There are some problems associated with the use of augmentative communication aids. These include:

1. speed of transmission
2. giving the user time to access and transmit messages
3. training the user and communicative partners to operate the device effectively
4. the social, cognitive, communication and physical needs of the user and potential communicative partners
5. the storage, capacity, size and portability of technical aids.

These are important factors when considering the usefulness of these devices in communicative interactions in general and when deciding upon their use by a person with a communication disability in particular.

Investigating the Use of a ScanWolf VOCA

To understand the impact of these issues on the use of a VOCA by a student with severe intellectual and multiple disabilities, a single subject case study was conducted in 1989. The study involved a 17-year-old male student in a special school in Canberra for secondary school students with severe intellectual disability. This student's communicative behaviour when using the ScanWolf VOCA was examined. Of special interest to this investigation were the student's initiations of communicative interactions and his responses and response modes (aided and unaided) to the communicative initiations of others, in terms of their frequency across three school settings. The settings used in this investigation were an advisory group (a semi-structured teacher-directed setting) and the recess and lunch breaks (unstructured settings).

Setting and Subject Description

The student selected for the case study attended a school catering for 120 students aged from 12 to 20 years, who have moderate to severe intellectual disability, many of whom have multiple disabilities. Each student's level of functioning, needs and potentials are unique, with functional levels ranging from total dependence on others through to a level allowing work placement in supported open employment.

Communication and language skills vary considerably within the student population. A total communication approach is used with all students, including those with functional verbal skills. Normal speech, manual signing, COMPIC symbols, functional reading and writing are everyday communication skills to which students are exposed.

Stephen, the subject of this study, was selected because of his particular communication needs. He has spastic quadriplegia associated with cerebral palsy and he also has an intellectual disability. Stephen has no oral language due to paralysis of the speech musculature. He suffers epilepsy resulting in petit mal seizures. He is confined to an electric wheelchair which he operates manually by pushing a joystick located close to his body on his wheelchair tray. Stephen had been using a symbol communication board attached to the wheelchair tray to communicate for some years. However, due to deterioration of his physical condition, his manual access to the board had become severely restricted, limiting his communicative activities. It became necessary, therefore, to investigate an alternative means of communication for him.

Research Design

The study took the form of a single-subject, multiple baseline across settings design to investigate the impact of the ScanWolf VOCA on Stephen's communicative interactional behaviour over three naturally occurring settings in the school. Communicative interactions were defined to include subject-initiated communication and the subject's responses to the communicative initiations of peers, school staff and others in the school. The multiple baseline across settings design is shown in Table 6-1.

Procedures

Establishing Stephen's readiness to use a portable electronic device in the form of a voice synthesiser as a communication aid was based on the following data. Information was obtained from school academic and medical files and through panel discussions involving the school's specialist speech/communication teacher, the computer teacher, the school counsellor, Stephen's advisory group teacher, the consultant occupational therapist and the physiotherapist, together with input from his parents.

Assessment was made of Stephen's current means of communication, including facial expression, eye and head movements, and direct access to the communication board using finger-pointing. His ability to use COMPIC symbols and simple written phrases was also established through the verbal and written reports of teachers, as his score on the Peabody Picture Vocabulary Test R was too low for reliable assessment. Visual and auditory skills were assessed together with his range of movement and scanning skills by the computer teacher and the consultant occupational therapist. Stephen's desire to communicate as well as his social skills were also evaluated by teaching staff and the specialist communication/speech teacher through the use of observation and checklists, as these areas are crucial to communicative behaviours.

Prior to the baseline phase, Stephen was given initial training in the use of the VOCA to establish an appropriate input-selection method and to familiarise him with operational procedures. The training period occurred over four half-hour sessions during one week. During that time, the vocabulary overlay was designed, on which 36 items, 6 per row, were displayed as COMPIC symbols, written single words and simple phrases relating to everyday functional and social life.

Table 6-1: Research design.

Setting	Week 1	Week 2	Week 3	Week 4
1. Advisory group	A	B	B	B
2. Recess	A	A	B	B
3. Lunch	A	A	A	B

Code: Condition A = Baseline; Condition B = Intervention.

This overlay also incorporated suggestions from Stephen, his parents and school staff.

The focus of measurement was on direct, observable communicative behaviours, that is, body and eye movements, facial expressions and direct usage of the communication board during baseline conditions and during the use of the ScanWolf VOCA. The frequencies of subject-initiated communicative interactions and subject responses to communicative initiations by others in each of the three school settings were observed and recorded by two observers operating simultaneously but independently of each other. Each observation session was of 15 minutes' duration in each of the three settings. They were conducted at the same time each day throughout baseline and intervention phases of the study. Inter-observer reliability checks were conducted during the baseline and intervention phases. Six reliability checks were made, one for each setting during baseline conditions and one for each of the settings during the intervention phase. Inter-observer agreement scores for the frequency data ranged between 90% and 100%.

During the baseline phase (Condition A in Table 6-1), communicative modes were identified in relation to Stephen's communicative initiations and responses. Observed modes of communication included head and eye movements, facial expressions and direct usage of a communication board containing single words, simple phrases and COMPIC symbols.

During the intervention phase (Condition B in Table 6-1), the ScanWolf VOCA replaced the manual communication board and was introduced systematically to each setting, that is, Week 2 in Setting 1, Week 3 in Setting 2 and Week 4 in Setting 3. Observed modes of communication were as for the baseline phase except for the change from communication board to the VOCA. Frequency data were collected as shown in Table 6-2.

Analyses of findings were made by visual inspection of graphed data leading to conclusions as to whether changes in communicative

Table 6-2: Data collection plan.

Condition	Observations
A. Baseline	4 × 15-minute sessions in advisory group 8 × 15-minute sessions in recess break 12 × 15-minute sessions in lunch break
B. Intervention	12 × 15-minute sessions in advisory group 8 × 15-minute sessions in recess break 4 × 15-minute sessions in lunch break

initiations and responses occurred over the three defined settings.

A staff questionnaire was also devised and trialled and was distributed to nine school staff members at the conclusion of the four-week study period. Respondents were those considered to be most familiar with Stephen in the school environment. The questionnaire was analysed in relation to staff perceptions of Stephen's communicative behaviours and self-esteem prior to and after the introduction of the ScanWolf VOCA.

Results

Figure 6-1 shows the frequency of Stephen's communicative initiations across the three school settings — advisory group, recess and lunch. Altogether, 16 × 15-minute observations were made in each setting, with a total of 48 × 15-minute observations made during the study. All settings were observed at baseline conditions for at least Week 1 of the study. The ScanWolf was introduced in Week 2 to the advisory group setting, in Week 3 to the recess setting and in Week 4 to the lunch setting.

Figure 6-1 does show a systematic increase in the frequency of Stephen's communicative initiations following the introduction of the ScanWolf VOCA to each setting. The data reveal a decrease in the number of initiations made by Stephen in the advisory group setting in the first week of intervention, while there was an increase in his initiations in recess and lunch breaks immediately following the introduction of the VOCA during the intervention phase. The decrease in the advisory group setting may have been due to the change from a traditional communication board to an electronic device and the need to use the novel device in a group situation. While Stephen had been given several training and familiarisation sessions in a one-to-one situation with the speech/communication teacher prior to the study, having to use the VOCA in an everyday situation with a group of peers and staff may have been disconcerting for him at first.

Figures 6-1 and 6-2 show that there is a small decrease in the number of initiations made by Stephen during recess and lunch in the Week 2 of those settings' baselines, coinciding with the introduction of the VOCA to the first setting, the advisory group. A similar result is shown for the lunch setting, coinciding with the introduction of the VOCA to the recess setting in Week 3. Data show an immediate increase in the number of Stephen's communicative initiations in recess and lunch breaks, coinciding with the introduction of the ScanWolf VOCA to those settings in Weeks 3 and 4. Stephen's communicative initiations in each week and for each phase and setting of the study are shown in Figure 6-2.

A total of 121 initiations were made by Stephen in the 48 × 15-

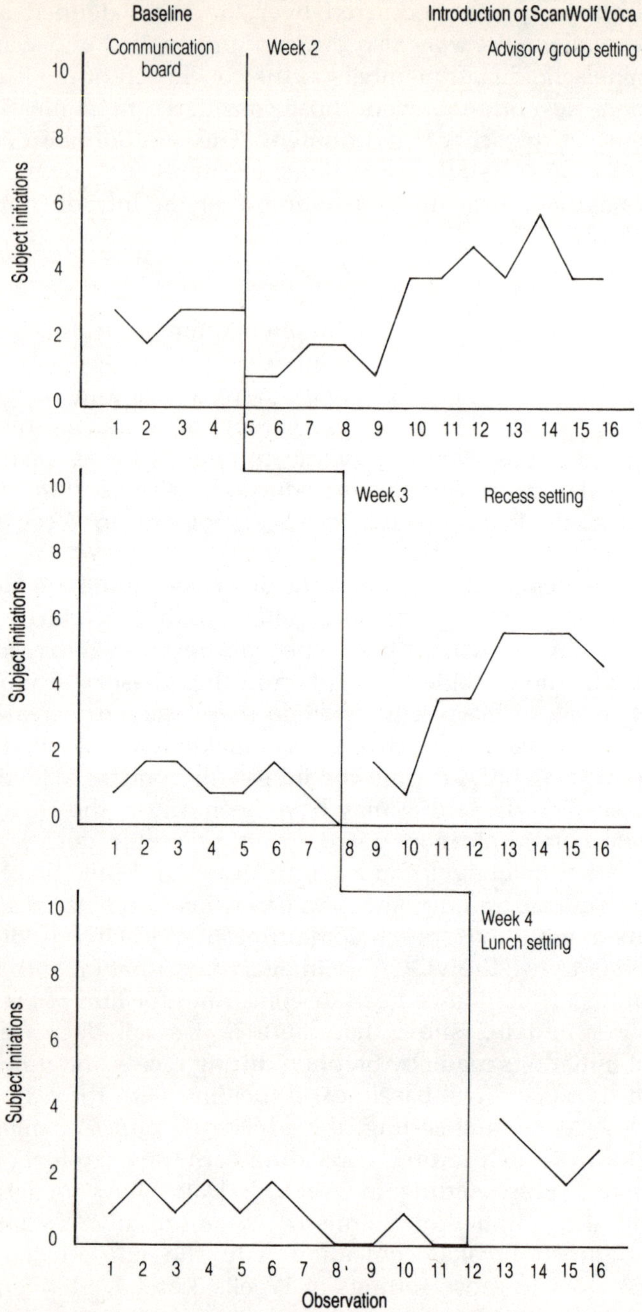

Figure 6-1: Frequency of subject-initiated communication over 16 × 15-minute observations for each setting.

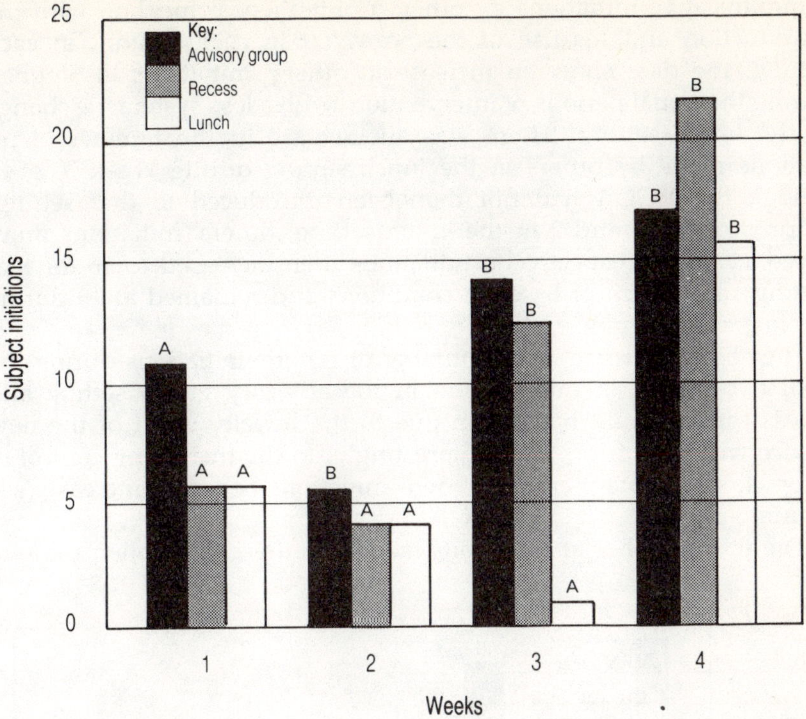

Figure 6-2: Weekly numbers of subject-initiated communicative interactions. Code: A = Baseline; B = Intervention.

minute observation sessions, 32 of which were made during the six baseline phase conditions and 89 of which were made during the six intervention phase conditions across the three settings.

The data reveal a large increase in the number of communicative initiations made by Stephen in the recess break. He made 10 initiations during 8 × 15-minute sessions in the baseline phase but 35 initiations over 8 × 15-minute sessions in the intervention phase.

In the lunch setting observations, the number of initiations increased by 15 when the VOCA was introduced. This substantial increase may possibly be explained as the result of Stephen's practice with the ScanWolf VOCA over the three weeks he was using it in the other two settings prior to the introduction of the ScanWolf to the lunch break in Week 4.

In summary, Figure 6-2 clearly indicates systematic increases in Stephen's communicative initiations with the introduction of the ScanWolf VOCA to each of the observation settings.

Data shown in Figure 6-3 reveal corresponding increases in the communicative initiations by others to Stephen, coinciding with the introduction and his use of the ScanWolf in each setting. In each setting, the data show an increase in others' initiations to Stephen during the initial periods of intervention, with a less systematic change in the lunch setting. There was an increase in the number of initiations made by others in the lunch setting during Week 3, even though the VOCA had not then been introduced to that setting. During Weeks 1 and 2 in the lunch setting, others' initiations numbered 11 and 6 respectively. Initiations then increased to 16 for that setting's last week of baseline conditions and remained at 16 during the intervention phase.

The slight decrease in the number of others' initiations during the final two weeks of intervention in the advisory group setting and recess setting could have been due to the novelty effect of the new device wearing off or, more interestingly, to the increasing control of interactions by Stephen as his own initiations began to increase (see Figure 6-2).

The total number of initiations made by others to Stephen came to

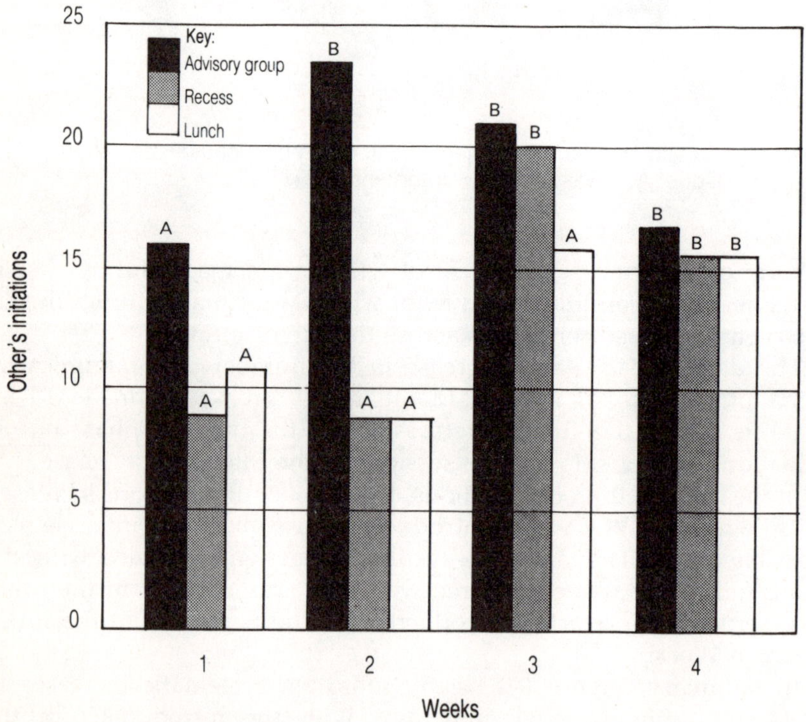

Figure 6-3: Communicative initiations made by others to the subject. Code: A = Baseline; B = Intervention.

186 initiations in the 48 × 15-minute observation sessions. Seventy-one initiations occurred during baseline conditions across the three settings, with 115 initiations occurring during intervention, showing an increase in the number of communicative initiations made by others once the VOCA was made available to Stephen to use.

Figure 6-4 shows a pattern of high non-vocal response to others by Stephen in the form of eye and head movements and facial expression when he used a communication board in responding to communication initiated by others during the baseline phase in all settings. However, the intervention phase data reported in Figure 6-4 also show that Stephen used his ScanWolf to respond to initiations more frequently than he used the communication board, while maintaining the non-vocal behaviour.

These data show a rise in non-vocal responses and a sharp decrease in the use of the ScanWolf to respond during the first three days of the ScanWolf intervention in the advisory group setting. This pattern coincides with that revealed in an analysis of Stephen's communication initiations at the same time in the same setting (see Figure 6-1), when his initiations also decreased for, presumably, the same reason.

Figure 6-5 shows the total number of non-vocal and aided communicative responses used by Stephen for each week, study phase and setting. Altogether 198 responses were made by Stephen to communicative initiations by others. Fourteen responses can be explained as being a conversational extension of the communicative exchange. Four of these extensions occurred in the advisory group setting in Week 3 of intervention, two non-vocal forms in the second week of baseline conditions during recess, two aided extensions in the first week of intervention during recess and one non-vocal extension in the second week of intervention during recess. Three non-vocal and two aided extensions occurred in the lunch setting during the baseline phase.

During the baseline phase, 77 responses were made by Stephen to 71 communicative initiations, and he made a total of 121 responses to 115 initiations by others during intervention conditions.

Non-vocal responses made during baseline conditions across the three settings numbered 64, or 83% of the total number of responses. The communication board was used 13 times, that is, 17% of the total number of responses to a total of 71 initiations.

During the intervention phase, the ScanWolf VOCA was used 64 times, or 52% of the total number of responses, and there were 57 non-vocal responses, that is, 47% of the time in response to a total of 115 initiations. Non-vocal communicative responses were used 83% of the time over baseline conditions compared to 47% during intervention. The use of aided modes of communication was 17% for the

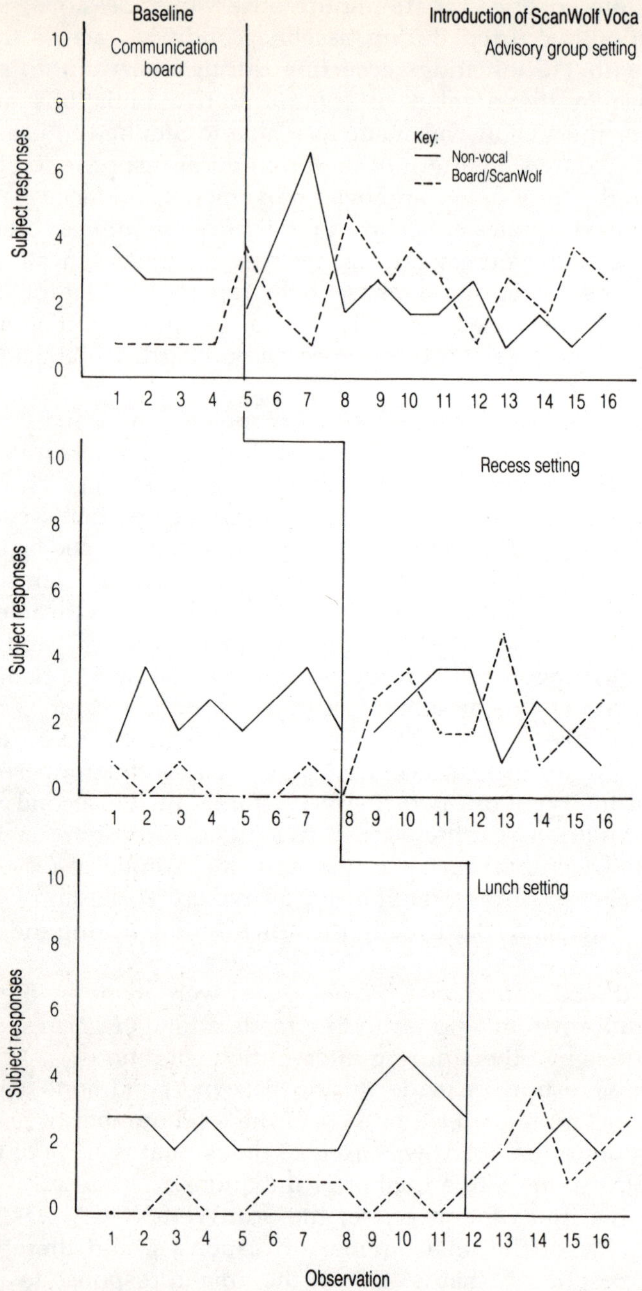

Figure 6-4: Frequency of the subject's responses, non-vocal and aided, to the communicative initiation of others.

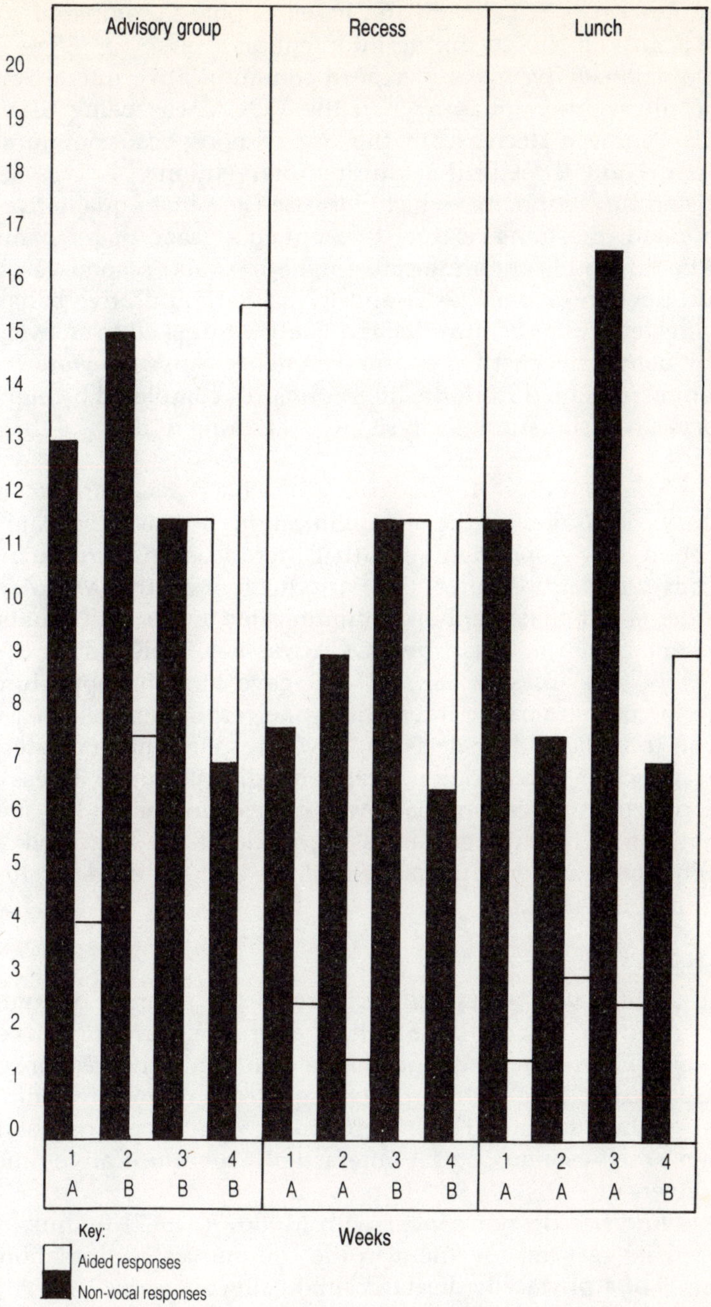

Figure 6-5: Numbers of non-vocal and aided communicative responses.

communication board during the baseline phase, compared to 52% for the ScanWolf VOCA during intervention.

These data clearly reveal increased communicative interaction during the intervention phase, when the VOCA was being used. The data also show a decrease in the use of non-vocal communicative forms across the three settings during intervention.

The staff questionnaire, which was used to obtain qualitative data, incorporated questions relating to Stephen's usage of his communication board, to his communicative initiations and responses prior to the introduction of the VOCA and to his communicative behaviours and self-esteem after its introduction. Staff were asked to answer questions by using checklist boxes and comments. Answers were collated and comments noted from the questionnaires completed by eight staff members. No statistical analysis was attempted due to the small sample.

There was a mixed result in the teachers' assessments of the frequency of usage of the communication board to initiate communication, but respondents felt that there was an increase in communicative initiations after the introduction of the VOCA. Most respondents felt that Stephen communicated more with adults than with peers. Seven felt that the VOCA was a suitable aid for Stephen as he now had access to an aid that gave him the opportunity to engage in communicative interaction; one respondent felt that it was too soon to make a clear decision. Seven respondents indicated that, due to muscular deterioration, Stephen's direct manual access to his traditional communication board was limited, inhibiting his ability to communicate. The different accessing mode of the ScanWolf VOCA had enhanced his communicative abilities and, as a result, his self-esteem had improved.

Discussion

The results indicate a marked increase in the number of communicative initiations made by Stephen after the introduction of the ScanWolf VOCA. The frequency of his communicative responses also increased, coinciding with an increase in communicative initiations made by others to him. There were strong indications from staff that Stephen's self-esteem, social interaction, communicative initiation and conversational skills had improved.

These findings do not concur with Molloy's (1987) findings which indicated no real improvement in the communicative initiations and responses of a physically disabled child using a Vocriss VOCA. However, Molloy concluded that the child was unable to become familiar with the device and that the size and lack of portability of the Vocriss did not offer access at all times. In the present study, Stephen was able to learn to use the ScanWolf VOCA in the four half-hour training sessions conducted before it was introduced into the school settings. In addition, the ScanWolf VOCA is a small, portable, battery-operated device, easily attached to a wheelchair tray, and has a single-switch activator providing the user with easy access at all times.

The findings of this study also do not confirm those of Calculator and Bollaghen (1982), Harris (1982) or Light, Collier and Parnes (1985), who asserted that children and adults with moderate to severe disabilities rarely used their augmentative aids to initiate communicative interaction. Those authors also concluded that the children and adults made few social comments and rarely requested information. While no analysis was made of the pragmatic functions of Stephen's utterances in this study, it was observed that he frequently used the VOCA to request information such as "What's happening?", "What are you doing?", and to offer assistance such as "Can I help?".

The present findings indicate that the ScanWolf facilitated an increase in the use of aided communication and a decrease in the use of non-vocal modes. Figures show that there was a marked increase in the usage of augmentative communication after the ScanWolf VOCA replaced the traditional communication board.

Importantly, the nature of this study puts certain limitations on the generalisations that might be made about the ScanWolf VOCA as a communication aid. The investigation was concerned with the communicative interactions, abilities and needs of a *single* student with individual-specific multiple deficits, attending a specific school environment. Its settings were based on a modified high school program in which students move from class to class and from teacher to teacher throughout the course of the school day. The VOCA was unable to be taken home with Stephen due to insurance restrictions, so observations were restricted to measuring his communicative interactions within the school grounds. These factors combined to prevent the generalisation of these findings to other individuals and settings.

Limitations in the use of the ScanWolf VOCA itself are significant. While it can be positioned easily on a wheelchair tray, allowing easy access to the single switch, the ScanWolf VOCA cannot be turned on and off by a single-switch user. Similarly, vocabulary overlays have to be changed by another person.

Concluding Comment

The assessment of a prospective user of an augmentative communication aid is vitally important. The range of physical movement, the ability to depress and release a switch, visual scanning abilities and auditory acuity must be established to ensure that the user has access to and can effectively operate the ScanWolf. The desire to communicate and the ability to understand and use functional language and to identify symbols, pictures and words are necessary for the student to be able to use the VOCA to advantage. A student who is already using a communication board effectively would, presumably, have these skills.

As with any augmentative communication aid, the time factor and the skills of potential communication partners are relevant. Scanning for and depressing the switch to activate the desired item takes time, so the communication partner must be prepared to wait. In a special school, not all students realise that they must wait for a response and, indeed, some staff must learn this skill too.

However, the results of this study do indicate that the use of a small portable device such as the ScanWolf VOCA can assist some students with severe communication difficulties and multiple disabilities to participate more fully in a learning and social environment and to develop a more positive self-image. Rather than being placed in a passive receiver role, the student can use the device to respond to and initiate discussion in class, in the playground, at home and in the community.

While augmentative communication systems do not solve all the communication problems a non-vocal person may experience and will not ensure effective communication (Calculator and Luchko, 1983; Shane & Bashir, 1980), the ScanWolf VOCA appeared to be more effective than the communication board in enhancing Stephen's communicative interactions and in giving him more control over his environment.

References

Austin, J.L. (1962). *How to do things with words*. London: Oxford University Press.

Bates, E. (1976). From gesture to first word: On cognitive and social prerequisites. In M. Lewis & L. Rosenblum (eds), *Origins of behavior: Language and communication*. N.Y.: John Wiley & Sons.

Bates, E., Camaoini, L. & Volterra, V. (1975). The acquisition of performatives prior to speech. *Merrill-Palmer Quarterly 21*, 205–26.

Bernstein, D.K. & Tiegerman, E. (1989). *Language and communication disorders in children*. Columbus, Ohio: Charles E. Merrill.

Beukelman, D. & Yorkston, K. (1977). A communicative system for the severely dysarthric speaker with an intact language system. *Journal of Speech and Hearing Disorders 42*, 265–70.

Bloom, L. & Lahey, M. (1982). *Language development and language disorders*. N.Y.: John Wiley & Sons.

Bloomberg, K. & Johnson, H. (1991). *Communication without speech*. Melbourne: ACER.

Boltorf, F.L. & De Pape, D. (1982). Initiating communication systems for severely speech impaired persons. *Topics in Language Disorders 2*, 55–72.

Calculator, S. & Dollaghen, C. (1982). The use of communication boards in a residential setting: An evaluation. *Journal of Speech and Hearing Disorders 47*, 281–87.

Calculator, S. & Luchko, C. (1983). Evaluating the effectiveness of a communication based program. *Journal of Speech and Hearing Disorders 48*, 185–91.

Chapman, R.S. & Miller, J.J. (1980). Analysing language and communication in the child. In R.L. Schiefelbusch (ed.), *Nonspeech language and communication: Analysis and intervention*. Baltimore: University Park Press.

Clarke, C. (1981). Learning words using traditional orthography and symbols of Rebus, Bliss and Carrier. *Journal of Speech and Hearing Disorders 46*, 191–96.

Duchan, J.F. (1984). Language assessment: The pragmatics revolution. In R.C. Naremore (ed.), *Language science*. San Diego: College Hill Press.

Halliday, M.A.K. (1975). *Explorations in the functions of language*. London: Arnold.

Harris, D. (1982). Communicative intervention processes involving non-vocal, physically handicapped children. *Topics in Language Disorders 2*, 21–38.

Harris, D. & Vanderheiden, G. (1980). Augmentative communication techniques. In R.L. Schiefelbusch (ed.), *Nonspeech language and communication: Analysis and intervention*. Baltimore: University Park Press.

Houghton, J., Bronicki, B. & Guess, D. (1987). Opportunities to express preferences and make choices among students with severe disabilities in classroom settings. *Journal of the Association for Persons with Severe Handicaps 12 (1)*, 18–27.

Kahn, J. (1977). A companion of manual and oral language training. *Mental Retardation 15*, 21–3.

Kraat, A. (1985). *Communication interaction between aided and natural speakers: A state of the art report*. Toronto: Rehabilitation Council for the Disabled.

Light, J., Collier, B. & Parnes, P. (1985). Communicative interaction between young, nonspeaking, physically disabled children and their primary caregivers (Part II: Communicative function). *Augmentative and Alternative Communication 11*, 98–107.

Lloyd, L. (1985). Comments on terminology. *Augmentative and Alternative Communication 1*, 95–7.

McLean, J.E. & Snyder-McLean, L. (1987). Form and function of communicative behaviour among persons with severe developmental disability. *Australia and New Zealand Journal of Developmental Disabilities 13*, 83–98.

Mirenda, P., Iacono, T. & Williams, R. (1990). Communication options for persons with severe and profound disabilities: State of the art and future directions. *Journal of the Association for Persons with Severe Handicaps 15*, 3–21.

Molloy, S. (1987). *An investigation into the introduction of the Vocriss, a synthesised voice output communicator, with a non-verbal child who has cerebral palsy*. Graduate Diploma dissertation. Submitted to Charles Sturt University-Mitchell, Bathurst, NSW.

Muma, J. (1978). *Language handbook*. Englewood Cliffs, NJ: Prentice-Hall.

Musselwhite, C.R. & St Louis, K.W. (1988). *Communication programming for persons with severe handicaps* (2nd edn). Boston: College Hill Press.

Nietupski, J. & Hamre-Nietupski, S. (1979). Teaching auxiliary communication skills to severely handicapped learners. *AAESPH Review* 4, 107–24.

Pitt, S. (1988). *Minspeak: Does it work?* Paper delivered to the Seventh Australasian Seminar of Technical Aid to the Disabled, Ryde, NSW.

Rees, N. (1978). Pragmatics of language: Application to normal and disordered language development. In R. Schiefelbusch (ed.), *Bases of language intervention*. Baltimore: University Park Press.

Schiefelbusch, R.L. (ed.) (1980). *Nonspeech language and communication: Analysis and intervention*. Baltimore: University Park Press.

Shane, H. & Bashir, A. (1980). Election criteria for the adoption of an augmentative communication system: Preliminary considerations. *Journal of Speech and Hearing Disorders 45*, 408–14.

Silverman, F. (1980). *Communication for the speechless*. Englewood Cliffs, NJ: Prentice-Hall.

Snell, M.E. (ed.) (1993). *Instruction of students with severe disabilities* (4th edn). Columbus, Ohio: Charles E. Merrill.

Vanderheiden, G.C. (ed.) (1978). *Non-vocal communication resource book*. Baltimore: University Park Press.

Vanderheiden, G.C. (1982). *Computers can plan a dual role for disabled individuals*. Madison, Wi: University of Wisconsin, Trace Center.

Vanderheiden, G.C. & Lloyd, L. (1986). Communication systems and their components. In S. Blackstone (ed.), *Augmentative communication: An introduction*. Rockville: American Speech-Language-Hearing Association.

Van Tatenhove, G. (1986). Transition through graphic symbol systems. *Communication Outlook 6 (3)*, 27–9.

Chapter 7

Communication Instruction in the 1990s: An Overview of Future Directions

Michael Arthur

University of Newcastle
Newcastle, NSW

Robert Williams, an American advocate for people with severe disabilities, recently published a powerful and timely call for a *communication imperative* (1991), in which he underlined the strategic importance and dignity of communicative growth for *all* individuals. He suggested a number of significant potential outcomes of such a movement, all of which hinge on the recognition of a need for change in both specific learning environments and the wider community, across the domains of knowledge, skills and attitudes. What, then, will such an imperative involve? What are its parameters? What part will instruction in educational contexts play? How can such change be achieved?

This chapter sets out to synthesise future directions for communication instruction in the 1990s, by identifying key findings in the research literature and integrating them with an ecological view of the communication process. A cyclical model is introduced and used as a basis for the analysis of a number of important themes. However, if Williams' urgent plea is to be translated into reality, this model must move from the status of best practice to that of general practice. As Calculator and Jorgensen noted recently (1991), it cannot be assumed that a knowledge of best practices will automatically result in their implementation. The linkage of principle to practice, then, and some points regarding the accompanying research agenda will be canvassed in the following pages.

At the outset, it is important to clarify our understanding of the term "communication". If speech can be typified as one *form* of communication, and language a *system* of signals designed to code our ideas about the world (McCormick & Schiefelbusch, 1990), then communication is the larger social *process* of informational exchange. Perhaps the most comprehensive definition is one adapted from the work of Dunst (1978, p 111), suggesting that communication is:

> . . . any overt conventional or non-conventional behavior, whether used intentionally or not, that has the effect of arousing in an onlooker a belief that the signal producing [person] is attempting to convey a message, make a demand, request, etc, to an onlooker.

What can be noted from this definition? Firstly, communication is interaction. This has important implications for both how and why we provide instruction to our students, as well as impacting on the social validity of communication instruction as an educational priority. Secondly, the range of behaviour acceptable as communicative is noteworthy. As suggested later, it is more than possible that the legacy of a historic focus on language skills in isolation has been the ignorance of much that is communicative in the people we seek to serve. Thirdly, communication, according to Dunst, can occur prior to the development of an intent to communicate. The facilitator of the learner's communicative behaviour, who may be a teacher, parent, therapist, aide or friend, "reads" the person's behaviour as communicative and shapes the form of the interaction. Finally, the process has contextual relevance. The message has meaning in and for the setting in which it occurs. If the many idiosyncratic forms of communication used by our students are interpreted positively and appropriately, the ability to make choices and take control of many elements of their lives (Williams, 1991) is within reach.

Throughout this discussion, the client group will be referred to interchangeably as students, learners or people with severe disabilities. This infers that these children and adults have an identified developmental disability, usually indicated by a score of 35 or less on a standardised intelligence test such as the *Stanford Binet Intelligence Scale*, 4th edition (Thorndike, Hagen & Sattler, 1986) or the *Wechsler Intelligence Scale for Children — Revised* (Wechsler, 1974), and significant deficits in adaptive behaviour as measured by an instrument such as the *Vineland Adaptive Behavior Scales* (Sparrow, Balla & Cicchetti, 1985).

Figure 7-1, below, proposes a dynamic view of communication in which interaction is linked across three dimensions: an individual's functional needs and learning processes, the immediate social context and the wider social context. This model will now be considered.

Individual Functioning: Needs and Learning Processes

Instruction in the Natural Setting

A great deal of research evidence and argument has accumulated to suggest that communication instruction is most effective when conducted in, and targeted at, the environments in which it is to be used (Goetz & Sailor, 1988; Halle, 1988; Norris & Hoffman, 1990; Romski, Lloyd & Sevcik, 1988). A general acceptance of the failure of the operant training approaches of the 1970s to promote learner spontaneity and skill generalisation led to the development of a number of new strategies in the 1980s, all of which centre on the *context of communication* as the key (see also Chapter 5 in this book). The questions of *where* and *when* instruction took place became integral to the construction of the instructional process, having a strong influence on *how* communication skills were taught. Examples of this new genre include mand-model techniques (Rogers-Warren & Warren, 1980), time delay (Schwartz, Anderson & Halle, 1989) and interrupted behaviour chains (Gee, Graham, Goetz, Oshima & Yoshioka, 1991). (For a full review of these and other related strategies, see Mirenda and Iacono, 1988).

The historic emphasis on the use of massed trials in artificial situations has been supplanted by a reliance, in many of these newer approaches, on the structured use, throughout the day and across environments and personnel, of naturally arising opportunities for interaction and instruction (Goetz & Sailor, 1988). This is not to suggest that established principles of learning, such as the utility of

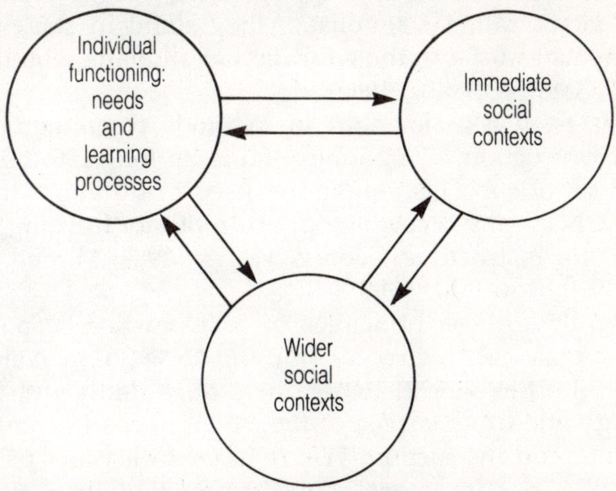

Figure 7-1: A cyclical view of communication processes relevant to the instruction of learners with severe disabilities.

cues, prompts and reinforcement, have been deserted. Rather, it is now accepted that the communication skills acquired by the learner are dependent upon the stimulus and reinforcement features of the wider environment in which the learner operates for generalised and spontaneous interaction to occur.

In a recent analysis, Halle (1987) introduced a continuum of controlling or discriminative stimuli relevant to spontaneity in learners with severe disabilities, and suggested that, at one extreme, factors such as the presence of a listener and contextual and interoceptive stimuli, such as hunger, can be directly linked to increased levels of spontaneous communication. Physical guidance, in contrast, provides a different locus of control and will result in decreased spontaneity.

In terms of generalisation effects, the instructional setting and what takes place within it have been hypothesised to be a powerful variable. Sailor, Goetz, Anderson, Hunt and Gee (1988) proposed a theory of context relevance in which they examined motivation effects across a number of dimensions. They argued that adjustments in the social environment of instruction will lead to improved learner abilities and interest in the acquisition and use of new communication skills. If, for example, a skill has immediate utility and practicality for a student, it can be expected to become generalised. Similarly, if a skill has a social base — that is, it is able to be used with more than one interactor — the likelihood of generalisation is increased. This point is of particular interest in light of the ever-increasing numbers of students who are moving into socially diverse and complex integrated settings (Brown, Schwarz, Udvari-Solner, Kampschroer, Johnson, Jorgensen & Gruenewald, 1991; Calculator & Jorgensen, 1991). Although these contextual factors appear simplistic, they stand in stark contrast to earlier approaches used in the education of students who have severe disabilities (Goetz & Sailor, 1988).

There has been a major shift in methods recommended for the delivery of instruction. Communication is no longer to be viewed as an isolated set of subskills taught and used in situations far removed from reality. Naturally occurring opportunities for learning must serve as the basis for instruction (Coots & Falvey, 1989; Mirenda, Iacono & Williams, 1990; Rowland, 1990).

How well have these principles of best practice been transferred into general practice? In a recent study in New South Wales (Arthur, Linfoot & Butterfield, 1992) 169 teachers of students with severe disabilities responded to a survey of their own needs in communication programming and instruction. When asked to list any techniques in communication enhancement or facilitation that they were familiar with or regularly used, only 4.7% ($n = 8$) identified items that could be categorised as "arranging the learning environment to enhance communicative interactions". Similarly, only 1.1% (n = 2) of the respondents indicated that they taught for generalisation. Although these figures are of a preliminary nature and concern an area that deserves future research attention, they do suggest that teachers are not necessarily implementing the types of strategies regarded as exemplary in the current literature. A recent publication, *Creating communicative contexts* (Butterfield, Arthur, Linfoot & Philips, 1992), is an attempt to address professional development needs in this area by providing a practical and responsive training program for school personnel.

The Functional Power of What is Learnt

Just as there has been a shift in the *where, when* and *how* of communication instruction, the content, or *what* is learnt, is now also very different to its earlier counterpart. Interventions of a decade or more ago focused on the descriptive or informational aspects of language, with less emphasis on the application or utility of this information (Goetz, Schuler & Sailor, 1981). More recently, researchers have been concerned with the pragmatic value of what is learnt. Much has been written about pragmatics in earlier chapters of this book. Burke (1990) described pragmatics as referring to the function of a behaviour and how it influences the environment, with particular reference to the effect that this has on regulating the behaviour of a listener. Examples include requests ("Want . . ."), rejections ("No want . . .") and greetings. As for context, attention has shifted to the interactive features of the communication process, a point which will be taken up a little later on in the discussion.

The functional role of communication raises many questions, all of which are relevant to content decisions. What can the learner do with this information? How effective is a particular concept or skill in increasing the independence and communicative power of a particular student? How can a functional analysis of a student's aberrant behaviour be used to select instructional content that is meaningful for the individual?

A number of researchers have provided evidence that students with severe disabilities do demonstrate a range of pragmatic functions in their interactive behaviour, in both structured and informal settings (Cirrin & Rowland, 1985; Linfoot, 1987). Of most recent interest has been the question of whether students with severe disabilities are primarily respondents, are dependent on others to begin and continue interactions, or whether they do in fact initiate communications at a level equivalent to their non-disabled peers (Kaczmarek, 1990; Romski, Sevcik, Reumann & Pate, 1989). In their 1987 study of the communicative life of 12 classrooms (37 students, 48 staff), Houghton,

Bronicki and Guess found that students with severe disabilities initiated interactions approximately once each minute, in both structured and unstructured situations.

Reichle, York and Eynon (1989) suggested that preference-indication (choice-making) is a particularly useful starting point for many learners, serving an instrumental purpose in the development of skills for initiating, maintaining and terminating interactions. As Guess, Benson and Siegel-Causey (1985) note, the ability to convey preferences is representative of personal autonomy and control over one's life. Thus, in terms of an if–then contingency, the learner begins to recognise why communication is important, as well as how to communicate, a concern raised by Gaylord-Ross and Holvoet (1985).

Additionally, the early work of Carr and Durand (1985), in identifying a sociocommunicative basis for aberrant behaviour within an operant paradigm, has led to the analysis of the communicative functions of behaviour and, conversely, the role of communication instruction as a means of decreasing or replacing inappropriate repertoires in learners with severe disabilities (Doss & Reichle, 1989). As Burke (1990) notes, recognising the purpose of a behaviour and providing assistance in the development of more appropriate means of expressing that purpose can be expected to result in decreased levels of frustration and antisocial behaviour. This view and the concomitant educational approach to behaviour change (Arthur, 1990; Evans & Meyer, 1985; Thompson, 1991) contrast with the traditional "eliminative" view of aberrant behaviour, criticised by Evans (1988), in which learning is dependent on and preceded by some form of behavioural readiness in the learner.

Recognising the Diversity of Communicative Behaviour

The field of augmentative and alternative communication has played a large part in the development of communicative competencies in individuals with severe disabilities (Musselwhite & St Louis, 1988). Technological support for communicative modes has been a major, arguably even the prime, contribution, often bridging the gap between an individual's drive to convey a message and the delivery of that message to a listener. However, as our definition of communication has broadened beyond the boundaries imposed by language, so the role of technology has changed. Two principles have accompanied this shift.

Firstly, communication must be viewed as a multimodal process. Although for many people speech is the primary form of communication, it is, without argument, supplemented by other perhaps less discernible and often idiosyncratic methods of exchange. Examples of these forms include changes in facial expressions, gestures, and gross movements of the body such as weight shifts. For some individuals, seemingly minor behaviours, such as eye flickers, or displays of pleasure, such as the conditional use of smiles, may play a large part in interactions with other people. Houghton et al (1987) identified a wide range of communicative behaviours in use in the classrooms they observed, with informal modes such as facial expressions most prevalent. In contrast, formal symbolic systems such as communication boards were the least often observed category. As suggested a little later, frequent and diverse communicative behaviours are of no functional value to the individual if the human environment in which they occur is non-responsive.

It is vital to recognise both the multiplicity of modes that are used and the fact that the sequence of modes demonstrated by any individual is ever-changing. A student may make a manually signed greeting upon arrival, vocalise when requested to place his or her bag in the corner and point to a preferred activity, all within the space of 30 seconds. Some researchers (Cirrin & Rowland, 1985; Reichle & Karlan, 1985) have suggested that the more successful communicators are those who have, and are encouraged to use, mixed modes of communication. Certainly, an inclusionary view of education must promote the acceptability of communicative diversity, rather than the reliance on one, and only one, means of communication. As Calculator (1988a, p 98) notes:

> Rather than placing differential value upon one mode of communication relative to another, instructional time might be better spent assisting individuals to use one or more modes, in various combinations, depending on the context.

Secondly, we must become adept at recognising the existing communication abilities of our students. As suggested earlier, for too long we have dismissed the preferences of some people whose behaviour is perceived to be aberrant (Williams, 1991) and failed to link interventions to the needs and desires of individuals to communicate (Baumgart, Johnson & Helmstetter, 1990). As an alternative, questions about the purpose of a behaviour should form the basis of our interventions. Similarly, conceptions of learner passivity may mask true communicative potential (Calculator, 1988b) and be influential in the development of learned helplessness (Seligman, 1975).

Thus, rather than arbitrarily selecting an augmentative system for a person and teaching him or her to master that system (Arthur, 1989; Kiernan, Reid & Jones, 1982), best practice commences with existing forms of communication and moves toward more universally "readable" modes that are appropriate for the individual (Arthur et al, 1992; Butterfield et al, 1992; Iacono, 1991).

Analysing How Learners Learn

Traditionally, the operant paradigm has guided the delivery and evaluation of communication instruction for learners with severe disabilities (Bowler, 1991). Essentially, the reasons for this can be attributed to the enormous empirical support for interventions that apply behavioural principles (Goetz & Sailor, 1988; Skiba & Casey, 1985).

Most recently, however, a number of researchers have proposed new directions which draw from the existing developmental and cognitive research literature. One such example is the movement-based approach of van Dijk (1986). Designed originally for students with dual sensory impairments, van Dijk's strategies are based on the early movement interactions evident in pre-language caregiver–infant relationships. Movement is viewed as a form of communication in which reciprocity is the key. An "action vocabulary" grounded in exchanges with a partner stimulates the learner's interest in the outside world and promotes increasing autonomous involvement with it. Siegel-Causey and Guess (1989), in their synthesis of practical strategies to enhance non-symbolic interactions, provide a profile of the approach and use scenarios to promote its integrated use in everyday contexts. Although the application of this approach to particular populations is in need of further controlled examination (Writer, 1987), two studies involving students with profound disabilities have provided encouraging preliminary results (Sternberg, Pegnatore & Hill, 1983; Sternberg, McNerney & Pegnatore, 1985). Further analyses will require tight control of confounding variables and longitudinal consideration of intervention effects.

Interestingly, a recent survey of teachers' perceptions of education and treatment needs for students with profound or multiple disabilities or medically fragile conditions (Izen & Brown, 1991) found that, of the 148 respondents, 40% regarded the van Dijk procedures/theory as often or very important. Conversely, 60% viewed this approach as not, or only occasionally, important. Of the teaching personnel who responded, 16.8% indicated that they included the approach in their classrooms, whilst 51.5% acknowledged that they didn't understand the term "van Dijk procedures". These findings will be of particular interest in the light of future research activity, by serving as a basis for comparisons with actual usage of the approach in educational programs.

Secondly, a recent attempt to meld the concerns of augmentative and alternative communication with those of the field of cognitive science will stimulate renewed interest in the broad question of how learners learn and, more specifically, the role of cognition in this process (Light & Lindsay, 1991). What is cognitive science, and how does it relate to communication instruction for students with severe disabilities? According to Johnson-Laird (1988, pp 26–7):

> The goal of cognitive science is to explain how the mind works . . . including some of the mind's most important tasks such as learning, remembering and communicating with others.

How do these tasks, and others involved in human learning, relate to the instructional needs of people with severe disabilities? The work by Mercer and Snell (1977), *Learning theory research in mental retardation: Implications for teaching*, is an excellent starting point for answering this question. Mercer and Snell critically examine a range of learning theories drawn from across the developmentalist–behaviourist continuum, and identify teaching implications for students with intellectual disabilities. Of particular interest is the presentation of a general learning paradigm which integrates, in a serial fashion, the following processes (1977, p 322):

1. expectancy: the influence of past experiences
2. selective attention: variations in learner attention to stimuli
3. input organisation: the coding of incoming information
4. memory: the retention and recall of information
5. transfer: generalising the usage of learnt material
6. performance: the outward demonstration of learning
7. feedback: information provided about responses made.

The difficulties a learner may have with any of these components serves as the rationale for intervention and remediation. While accepting many of the steps proposed by Mercer and Snell, a modern cognitive (information-processing) theory of learning, such as that espoused by Gagne (1975) and Gagne, Briggs and Wager (1988), is especially concerned to evaluate the internal thinking processes occurring in the learner. Although the role of the environment is acknowledged, cognitive scientists are particularly interested in the construction of theoretical models that can explain and account for how the mind deals with and responds to incoming information (Light & Lindsay, 1991).

In terms of communication instruction, then, there are many unresolved issues. How do naturalistic strategies, such as those discussed earlier, impact on what is occurring in a learner's mind? How influential will behavioural principles of instruction be, as new and divergent approaches are evaluated (Goetz & Sailor, 1988)? Is performance of a communication skill our only valid measure of its attainment? How do metacognitive (or thinking about our thinking) processes influence how we teach functional communication, and the related usage issues of maintenance and generalisation? These questions and many others like them will dominate the research agenda of the 1990s.

This section has identified and discussed a number of issues related to the communication instruction needs and learning processes of individuals with severe disabilities. To stop here, however, would be to leave the subject of communication instruction incomplete. As indicated in Figure 7-1, communication is by definition a social process, in which the human environment plays a pivotal role in the exercise of individual skills and the achievement of interaction. In essence, it is pointless being able to speak, sign, gesticulate or scan symbols on an augmentative communication system unless someone in your immediate environment is able and willing to interact with you. It is to this subject that our attention now turns.

Immediate Social Contexts

Improving the Responsiveness of Communicative Partners

The disturbing findings of Houghton et al (1987) have stimulated a great deal of interest in the ecology of communication. In this applied study of classroom interactions, staff were shown to be responding to student-initiated communications on only 7 to 15% of occasions. Furthermore, 99% of staff-initiated communications were followed by student responses. What do these findings tell us? Put simply, a great deal of the students' communicative behaviour was ignored. On a large number of occasions, staff appeared unable to recognise or respond to the initiatives of their students. The students who were observed, however, very rarely failed to respond when staff initiated an interaction. The potential outcomes of such a situation are manifold.

Firstly, faulty staff perceptions about the non-communicative status of their students may produce a downward spiral in terms of expectations. A number of writers (Calculator, 1988a; Mittler & Berry, 1977; Owings & Guyette, 1982) have suggested that partner anticipation of needs and wants can lead to underfunctioning by the learner. That is, the learner fails to behave in ways that may be expected, due to a perception that interaction is no longer necessary. Munson, Nordquist and Thuma-Rew (1987), in discussing the reliance of many students on partner direction of interactions, despite the presence of an augmentative or alternative system, concluded that partners' low expectations, as well as a history of failure in communication, are important explanatory factors. Secondly, and related to the preceding point, this imbalance promotes an "us–them" attitude to communication processes, rather than encouraging the development of a rich and balanced culture of interaction. Thirdly, the frustration caused by a lack of partner response may result in the demonstration of behaviours deemed to be inappropriate, thus potentially isolating the individual from a full and inclusive range of educational opportunities. Finally, the affective implications for students must be considered. Initial perceptions of powerlessness can be expected, over time, to give way to conditions of learned helplessness, in which an individual's motivation and general emotional state are guided by the belief that nothing they do counts (Seligman, 1975). The affective functioning of people with severe disabilities is one area where future research is particularly necessary.

What has been done, then, to address this situation? Mirenda et al (1990) call for the development of educational training programs for facilitators, to improve their knowledge of communication opportunities and modes. This author contends that such interventions must be even more inclusive, since knowledge in isolation is useless. All personnel who interact with people who have severe disabilities must receive structured assistance in the refinement of skills, knowledge and attitudes, and be able to recognise the overlap of these factors in practice. Families and, in particular, siblings are one subgroup whose needs in this area deserve further examination. These issues have high priorities in the field as we move through the 1990s.

Three recently published research reports are of relevance to this discussion. In the first (Haring et al, 1987), three teachers were trained in the use of four modified incidental-teaching procedures (such as blocking access, offering out-of-context objects and so on). The training was achieved by the teachers using a self-instruction manual and planning activities. Both teachers and students demonstrated skill improvements. As pointed out by the researchers, a number of design limitations, such as the lack of follow-up, tempers the raw findings. In particular, a longitudinal analysis of independent teacher behaviour is needed to validate genuine intervention effects. The study does represent, however, an important attempt to modify both student and teacher behaviour.

The second study (Schwartz, Anderson & Halle, 1989) used a multiple-baseline design to evaluate the effects of systematic training (explanation, role-playing and feedback) on both the use of opportunities for time delay by the teacher and student language usage. In summary, teachers mastered the use of the time delay procedure (thus increasing the number of student utterances) but needed further assistance before they were able to independently identify new opportunities for using the strategy. The researchers concluded that further work is needed to ensure teacher generalisation of learnt skills to situations in which there is no experimental "prompt".

In the third project (McNaughton & Light, 1989), facilitators were involved in the entire process of developing communication opportunities and participation support for a 27-year-old woman with severe intellectual disability. This holistic approach to staff training included the staff being responsible for the assessment, goal-setting and evaluation procedures used as well as for staff instruction in a range of interaction strategies. Although extremely limited by the case study design and anecdotal nature of the data reported, this model has much to recommend it. The facilitators are involved in, and empowered by, the whole planning process. It could be expected that they would take on ownership of, and responsibility for, both improvements in the learner's communicative competence and their own responsiveness. In particular, this approach encourages change across three fundamental domains (knowledge, skills and attitudes) by immersing the facilitator in a range of experiences all of which are interactive and relevant to naturally occurring situations. Additionally, the whole team (including day program and group home staff) were involved in the intervention.

A recent publication by Butterfield et al (1992), designed for staff in schools but appropriate to communication facilitators in a variety of settings, takes a similar broad-ranging view of training. Using a self-instruction manual, staff are provided with a practical process to follow in establishing communication assessment, programming and instructional procedures for their students. Emphasis is placed on the forms, functions and social components of communication. Of particular interest, however, is a staff rating scale which can be used to set personal goals, thereby raising awareness of the reciprocal nature of true communication. By scoring each item as either (1) often, (2) sometimes or (3) rarely, staff simply respond to the question "When you are with (Student) do you . . . ?":

1. look for opportunities to promote interaction
2. encourage shared focus on activities or objects
3. pace routines to allow for interactions
4. indicate that you expect the student to respond
5. acknowledge attempts to communicate and respond
6. provide opportunities for choice making
7. talk to the student about routines as they occur
8. avoid anticipating needs
9. respond to the students' initiatives and avoid frustration
10. provide adequate time for students to respond.

Future research must focus on optimal models of staff and parent training (McNaughton & Light, 1989) to identify ways in which generalised and applied change in communication environments can be achieved. If the Houghton et al (1987) study were to be replicated in 1997, it is hoped that there would be significant positive changes in staff behaviour. How to achieve this continues to attract debate. One important variable is interdisciplinary involvement and service delivery, particularly in the context of the burgeoning integration movement.

Integrating Service Delivery

Communication instruction for students with severe disabilities faces many new challenges as increasing numbers of individuals are, pleasingly, educated in regular settings (Williams, Villa, Thousand & Fox, 1989). The face of the immediate social context for many students, therefore, is changing. One method of positively influencing the quality of educational outcomes generally and, for this discussion, the outcomes of communication instruction in particular is the integration of related services (Meyer, Eichinger & Park-Lee, 1987; Sailor, Gee, Goetz & Graham, 1988; York & Rainforth, 1989). Essentially, this process calls for the development of a team approach, a partnership between members of various disciplines (such as speech pathology and teaching) for educational programming and delivery. The resulting integrated objectives (Calculator & Jorgensen, 1991) focus on the development of functional learner skills in environments that are receptive, unified and normalised.

How is a student's communicative context enhanced by integrated service delivery? Firstly, the presence of one intervention plan, achieved through consultation (Janney & Meyer, 1990), encourages uniform expectations and goals. Secondly, everybody interacting with the student is a potential facilitator of communication (Calculator & Jorgensen, 1991), in contrast with a traditional segmentation of roles. Thirdly, the context of the communication drives the interaction, with a variety of staff responding to naturally arising opportunities rather than an artificial reliance on one, and only one instructor, setting and methodology. In this way, a person assisting a student to eat a meal will look for ways to stimulate and expand upon student initiatives, in light of agreed objectives and evaluation techniques.

As an emerging framework for policy and practice, integrated service delivery is subject to constant analysis and re-formation. Giangreco (1990) identified the difficulties of coordination and decision-making in the field, especially as applied to roles, decision criteria and authority structures. He flagged the need for in-service education, administrative guidelines, changes in tertiary training programs and continuing research interest. Similarly, Dunn (1991, p 369) has called for the "establishment of administrative mechanisms that support integrated programming". York, Rainforth and Dunn (1990) have argued that the pre-service and ongoing training experiences of professionals working with people who have severe disabilities must reflect cross-disciplinary curricula to promote effective integration in service delivery. To date, this is an uncommon practice in most universities (Calculator & Jorgensen, 1991), a problem that, in this author's view, must be resolved before integrated service delivery can be fully effective.

This discussion has centred on the role of the immediate social context in communication instruction and has identified a number of important areas for development as the decade unfolds. In the final section of this chapter, some of the wider processes that impinge upon communication instruction are presented and discussed, guided by the notion that the communicative power of an individual is ultimately shaped by the recognition afforded him or her by society in general.

Wider Social Contexts

Improving Societal Inclusion

In a recent longitudinal study involving 91 students all of whom had severe or profound disabilities, Cole and Meyer (1991) showed that individuals who were integrated into regular settings progressed in demonstrated levels of social competence, while those who attended segregated schools regressed on the same measures. While it is not the intention of this author to survey the specifics of the integration debate here (Brown, Long, Udvari-Solner, Schwarz, Van-Deventer, Ahlgren, Johnson, Gruenewald & Jorgensen, 1989; Brown et al, 1991; Williams et al, 1989), it is important to note both the ongoing move toward regular education for all and the increasing empirical evidence for the efficacy of such an approach (Brinker & Thorpe, 1984; Cole & Meyer, 1991).

These points suggest, then, that in broad educational provisions society appears to be slowly progressing toward a more integrated and accepting approach to the needs of people with severe disabilities. In terms of communication, however, what does the future hold? Outside the school gates, how does the community at large view the communicative functioning of such individuals? Mirenda et al (1990) detailed a myriad of ways in which discrimination generally makes an impact upon specific aspects of the communication processes of these people. Examples of this deliberate or ignorant behaviour in society may range from teasing at the corner store as a person points to a preferred item, right through to a person being denied leisure opportunities because a bureaucrat cannot accept that such individuals are capable of enjoying themselves or communicating with others.

There is much to be done. Mirenda and her colleagues (1990, p 5) argue that, in addition to replacing ignorance with knowledge, we must identify the discriminatory factors in society that limit communication opportunities for people with severe disabilities and put into place responsive programs, such as "environmental reconstruction, awareness education and sensitization, advocacy and legislative efforts, and/or curricular and placement changes". One complementary strategy may be the adoption of a concerns-based approach to change. Following such an approach, remedial interventions, as Mirenda et al (1990) call them, can be based on and designed to address the very concerns or fears that the target group identifies as relevant to them. In this way, *real* as opposed to *perceived* needs are met.

Enhancing and Maintaining Social Networks

Communication is at the very heart of human relationships. Ultimately, we learn to communicate so that we can express ourselves, interact with others and exercise some control over our lives. The presence of a listener (or interactor) is one of the prerequisites of effective communication (Kaczmarek, 1990) and is something usually taken for granted by many of us. Indeed, for most people, communicative functioning and social functioning are complementary processes, influencing and relying upon each other.

In their recent study, Kennedy, Horner and Newton (1989) examined, over two and a half years, the social interaction patterns of 23 adults with severe disabilities living in the community. They showed that the social networks of their subjects were quite heavily dependent on family members and subject to high turnover. That is, maintenance of relationships was difficult. "It was unusual for a friend or acquaintance to continue to have contact with a participant for more than 1 year" (p 194). As the authors pointed out, the fact that the participants were living in atypical support settings (with better than average staffing ratios, for example) may have improved their social interaction patterns. Therefore, the typical situation for many people may well be worse than the one described in this study. Although this project was concerned with quantitative factors rather than any qualitative measure of social contacts, the implications for such people's communication processes are clear. Regardless of whether or not the presence of poor communication skills is a predictor of low durability in social relationships (a point that is presently unclear), it may be hypothesised that the difficulty of constantly changing companions will not serve to enhance functional communication skills in an individual. If a person with a severe disability does not have the opportunity to build a meaningful, long-term and truly communicative relationship with a partner or partners, apart from those who are paid to provide care, his or her aspirations and feelings of purpose may be adversely affected.

A great deal of research is needed to identify the links between social networking, communicative development and quality of life in general. In addition, we need to evaluate the types of interaction patterns in evidence. Do people with severe disabilities demonstrate a preference for socialisation with people who have similar disabilities, as is common among deaf people, or do they prefer more heterogeneous social relationships? Does a choice exist, or are networks imposed unilaterally? What part does communicative competence play in the socialisation process, and how can societal structures be changed to promote autonomy (C. Gordon, 22 February 1992, personal communication)?

Summary and Conclusions

In this chapter, future directions for communication instruction have been couched in terms of a dynamic three-component model. Implicit in the discussion has been the premise that communication as a phenomenon cannot exist in isolation. It has been argued that the skills a person develops are only of value when viewed from an ecological perspective. Ann Kaiser (1990), in her first editorial for the *Journal of The Association for Persons with Severe Handicaps,* emphasised the importance of an interactive view of research, within which the needs of the individual are contextualised.

Although many questions have been broached, their underlying theme has been consistent: the need to continue closing the gap between research and practice. In a very real sense, when it comes to communication, every one of us is a learner, whether we are trying to explain educational jargon, indicate our favourite food or advocate major policy change in disability legislation.

Bob Williams is right. We need a communication imperative!

References

Arthur, M. (1989). Augmentative communication systems for learners with severe disabilities: Towards effective assessment and placement practices. *Australia and New Zealand Journal of Developmental Disabilities 15 (2),* 119–25.

Arthur, M. (1990). *The impact of instruction and skill development on aberrant behaviour: The classroom reality.* Paper presented at the 26th National Conference of the Australian Society for the Study of Intellectual Disability, Adelaide.

Arthur, M., Linfoot, K. & Butterfield, N. (1992). *Concerns for best practice in communication interventions: An Australian study.* Manuscript submitted for publication.

Baumgart, D., Johnson, J. & Helmstetter, E. (1990). *Augmentative and alternative communication systems for persons with moderate and severe disabilities.* Baltimore: Paul H. Brookes.

Bowler, D.M. (1991). Need for theory in studies of augmentative and alternative communication. *Augmentative and Alternative Communication 7 (2)*, 127–32.

Brinker, R.P. & Thorpe, M.E. (1984). Integration of severely handicapped students and the proportion of IEP objectives achieved. *Exceptional Children 51*, 168–75.

Brown, L., Long, E., Udvari-Solner, A., Schwarz, P., Van-Deventer, P., Ahlgren, C., Johnson, F., Gruenewald, L. & Jorgensen, J. (1989). Should students with severe intellectual disabilities be based in regular or in special education classrooms in home schools? *Journal of The Association for Persons with Severe Handicaps 14 (1)*, 8–13.

Brown, L., Schwarz, P., Udvari-Solner, A., Kampschroer, E., Johnson, F., Jorgensen, J. & Gruenewald, L. (1991). How much time should students with severe intellectual disabilities spend in regular education classrooms and elsewhere? *Journal of The Association for Persons with Severe Handicaps 16 (1)*, 39–47.

Burke, G.M. (1990). Unconventional behavior: A communicative interpretation in individuals with severe disabilities. *Topics in Language Disorders 10 (4)*, 75–85.

Butterfield, N., Arthur, M., Linfoot, K. & Philips, S. (1992). *Creating communicative contexts: An instructional manual for teachers of students with severe intellectual disability*. Sydney: NSW Department of School Education.

Calculator, S.N. (1988a). Promoting the acquisition and generalization of conversational skills by individuals with severe handicaps. *Augmentative and Alternative Communication 4*, 94–103.

Calculator, S.N. (1988b). Teaching functional communication skills to adults with mental retardation. In S.N. Calculator & J. Bedrosian (eds), *Communication assessment and intervention for adults with mental retardation* (pp 309–38). San Diego: College-Hill Press.

Calculator, S.N. & Jorgensen, C.M. (1991). Integrating AAC instruction into regular education settings: Expounding on best practices. *Augumentative and Alternative Communication 7 (3)*, 204–14.

Carr, E.G. & Durand, V.M. (1985). The social-communicative basis of severe behavior problems in children. In S. Reiss & R. Bootzin (eds), *Theoretical issues in behavior therapy*. New York: Academic Press.

Cirrin, F. & Rowland, C. (1985). Communicative assessment of nonverbal youths with severe/profound mental retardation. *Mental Retardation 23*, 52–62.

Cole, D.A. & Meyer, L.H. (1991). Social integration and severe disabilities: A longitudinal analysis of child outcomes. *The Journal of Special Education 25 (3)*, 340–51.

Coots, J. & Falvey, M.A. (1989). Communication skills. In M.A. Falvey, *Community-based curriculum: Instructional strategies for students with severe handicaps* (2nd edn.). Baltimore: Paul H. Brookes.

Doss, S. & Reichle, J. (1989). Establishing communicative alternatives to the emission of socially motivated excess behavior: A review. *Journal of The Association for Persons with Severe Handicaps 14 (2)*, 101–12.

Dunn, W. (1991). Integrated related services. In L.H. Meyer, C.A. Peck & L. Brown (eds), *Critical issues in the lives of people with severe disabilities*. Baltimore: Paul H. Brookes.

Dunst, C.J. (1978). A cognitive-social approach for assessment of early non-verbal communicative behavior. *Journal of Childhood Communication Disorders 2*, 110–23.

Evans, I. (1988). *Non-aversive intervention for behavior problems*. Paper presented at the Macquarie University Behavior Management Conference, Sydney.

Evans, I. & Meyer, L.H. (1985). *An educative approach to behavior problems: A practical decision model for interventions with severely handicapped learners*. Baltimore: Paul H. Brookes.

Gagne, R.M. (1975). *Essentials of learning for instruction*. New York: Holt, Rinehart and Winston.

Gagne, R.M., Briggs, L.J. & Wager, W.W. (1988). *Principles of instructional design* (3rd edn). New York: Holt, Rinehart and Winston.

Gaylord-Ross, R. & Holvoet, J. (1985). *Strategies for educating students with severe handicaps*. Boston: Little Brown.

Gee, K., Graham, N., Goetz, L., Oshima, G. & Yoshioka, K. (1991). Teaching students to request the continuation of routine activities by using time delay and decreasing physical assistance in the context of chain interruption. *Journal of The Association for Persons with Severe Handicaps 16 (3)*, 154–67.

Giangreco, M.F. (1990). Making related service decisions for students with severe disabilities: Roles, criteria and authority. *Journal of The Association for Persons with Severe Handicaps 15 (1)*, 22–31.

Goetz, L. & Sailor, W. (1988). New directions: Communication development in persons with severe disabilities. *Topics in Language Disorders 8 (4)*, 41–54.

Goetz, L., Schuler, A. & Sailor, W. (1981). Functional competence as a factor in communication instruction. *Exceptional Education Quarterly 2*, 51–61.

Gordon, C. (1992). Personal communication. Communication seminars, Charles Sturt University-Mitchell.

Guess, D., Benson, H.A. & Siegel-Causey, E. (1985). Concepts and issues related to choice-making and autonomy among persons with severe disabilities. *Journal of The Association for Persons with Severe Handicaps 10 (2)*, 79–86.

Halle, J.W. (1987). Teaching language in the natural environment: An analysis of spontaneity. *Journal of The Association for Persons with Severe Handicaps 12 (1)*, 28–37.

Halle, J.W. (1988). Adopting the natural environment as the context of training. In S.N. Calculator & J. Bedrosian (eds), *Communication assessment and intervention for adults with mental retardation*. San Diego: College-Hill Press.

Haring, T.G., Neetz, J.A., Lovinger, L., Peck, C. & Semmel, M.I. (1987). Effects of four modified incidental teaching procedures to create opportunities for communication. *Journal of The Association for Persons with Severe Handicaps 12 (3)*, 218–26.

Houghton, J., Bronicki, G.J.B. & Guess, D. (1987). Opportunities to express preferences and make choices among students with severe disabilities in classroom settings. *Journal of The Association for Persons with Severe Handicaps 12 (1)*, 18–27.

Iacono, T. (1991). *Communication for children with severe intellectual disabilities*. Paper presented at the Fourth Annual Conference in Special Education, Charles Sturt University-Mitchell, Bathurst, NSW.

Izen, C.L. & Brown, F. (1991). Education and treatment needs of students with profound, multiply handicapping, and medically fragile conditions: A survey of teachers' perceptions. *Journal of The Association for Persons with Severe Handicaps 16 (2)*, 94–103.

Janney, R.E. & Meyer, L.H. (1990). A consultation model to support integrated educational services for students with severe disabilities and challenging behaviors. *Journal of The Association for Persons with Severe Handicaps 15 (3)*, 186–99.

Johnson-Laird, P.N. (1988). *The computer and the mind: An introduction to cognitive science*. Cambridge, MA: Harvard University Press.

Kaczmarek, L.A. (1990). Teaching spontaneous language to individuals with severe handicaps: A matrix model. *Journal of The Association for Persons with Severe Handicaps 15 (3)*, 160–69.

Kaiser, A.P. (ed.) (1990). Editorial: JASH in the 1990s. *Journal of The Association for Persons with Severe Handicaps 15 (1)*, 1–2.

Kennedy, C.H., Horner, R.H. & Newton, J.S. (1989). Social contacts of adults with severe disabilities living in the community: A descriptive analysis of relationship patterns. *Journal of The Association for Persons with Severe Handicaps 14 (3)*, 190–96.

Kiernan, C., Reid, B. & Jones, L. (1982). *Signs and symbols: A review of literature and survey of the use of non-vocal communication systems*. London: Academic Press.

Light, J. & Lindsay, P. (1991). Cognitive science and augmentative and alternative communication. *Augmentative and Alternative Communication 7 (3)*, 186–203.

Linfoot, K. (1987). *Communicative behaviour in children with severe developmental delay*. Unpublished doctoral dissertation. Sydney: Macquarie University.

McCormick, L. & Schiefelbusch, R.L. (1990). *Early language intervention: An introduction* (2nd edn). Columbus, Ohio: Charles E. Merrill.

McNaughton, D. & Light, J. (1989). Teaching facilitators to support the communication skills of an adult with severe cognitive disabilities: A case study. *Augmentative and Alternative Communication 5*, 35–41.

Mercer, C.D. & Snell, M.E. (1977). *Learning theory research in mental retardation: Implications for teaching*. Columbus, Ohio: Charles E. Merrill.

Meyer, L., Eichinger, J. & Park-Lee, S. (1987). A validation of program quality indicators in educational services for students with severe disabilities. *Journal of The Association for Persons with Severe Handicaps 12*, 251–63.

Mirenda, P. & Iacono, T. (1988). Strategies for promoting augmentative and alternative communication in natural contexts with students with autism. *Focus on Autistic Behaviour 3 (4)*, 1–16.

Mirenda, P., Iacono, T. & Williams, R. (1990). Communication options for persons with severe and profound disabilities: State of the art and future directions. *Journal of Thc Association for Persons with Severe Handicaps 15 (1)*, 3–21.

Mittler, P. & Berry, P. (1977). Demanding language. In P. Mittler (ed.), *Research to practice in mental retardation (vol. 2): Education and training*. Baltimore: University Park Press.

Munson, J., Nordquist, C. & Thuma-Rew, S. (1987). *Communication systems for persons with severe neuromotor impairment*. Iowa City: University of Iowa.

Musselwhite, C.R. & St Louis, K.W. (1988). *Communication programming for persons with severe handicaps: Vocal and augmentative strategies* (2nd edn). Boston: College-Hill Press.

Norris, J. & Hoffman, P. (1990). Language intervention within naturalistic environments. *Language, Speech and Hearing Services in Schools 21*, 72–84.

Owings, N. & Guyette, T. (1982). Communication behavior assessment and treatment with the adult: An approach. In N. Lass (ed.), *Speech and language: Advances in basic research and practice* (vol. 7). New York: Academic Press.

Reichle, J. & Karlan, G. (1985). The selection of an augmentative system in communication intervention: A critique of decision rules. *Journal of The Association for Persons with Severe Handicaps 10*, 146–56.

Reichle, J., York, J. & Eynon, D. (1989). Influence of indicating preferences for initiating, maintaining, and terminating interactions. In F. Brown & D.H. Lehr (eds), *Persons with profound disabilities: Issues and practices*. Baltimore: Paul H. Brookes.

Rogers-Warren, A. & Warren, S. (1980). Mands for verbalization: Facilitating the display of newly trained language in children. *Behavior Modification 4*, 361–82.

Romski, M.A., Lloyd, L.L. & Sevcik, R.A. (1988). Augmentative and alternative communication issues. In R.L. Schiefelbusch & L.L. Lloyd (eds), *Language perspectives* (2nd edn). Austin, Texas: Pro-Ed.

Romski, M.A., Sevcik, R.A., Reumann, R. & Pate, J.L. (1989). Youngsters with moderate or severe mental retardation and severe spoken language impairments 1: Extant communicative patterns. *Journal of Speech and Hearing Disorders 54*, 366–73.

Rowland, C. (1990). Communication in the classroom for children with dual sensory impairments: Studies of teacher and child behavior. *Augmentative and Alternative Communication 6*, 262–74.

Sailor, W., Gee, K., Goetz, L. & Graham, N. (1988). Progress in educating students with the most severe disabilities: Is there any? *Journal of The Association for Persons with Severe Handicaps 13 (2)*, 87–99.

Sailor, W., Goetz, L., Anderson, J., Hunt, P. & Gee, K. (1988). Research on community intensive instruction as a model for building functional generalized skills. In R. Horner, G. Dunlap & R. Koegel (eds), *Generalization and maintenance: Life style changes in applied settings*. Baltimore: Paul H. Brookes.

Schwartz, I.S., Anderson, S.R. & Halle, J.W. (1989). Training teachers to use naturalistic time delay: Effects on teacher behavior and on the language use of students. *Journal of The Association for Persons with Severe Handicaps 14 (1)*, 48–57.

Seligman, M. (1975). *Helplessness: On depression, development and death*. San Francisco: W.H. Freeman.

Siegel-Causey, E. & Guess, D. (1989). *Enhancing nonsymbolic communication interactions among learners with severe disabilities*. Baltimore: Paul H. Brookes.

Skiba, M.J. & Casey, A. (1985). Interventions for behavior disordered students: A quantitative review and methodological critique. *Behavioral Disorders 10*, 239–52.

Sparrow, S.S., Balla, D.A. Cicchetti, D.V. (1985). *Vineland Adaptive Behavior Scales*. Circle Pines: American Guidance Service, Inc.

Sternberg, L., McNerney, C.D. & Pegnatore, L. (1985). Developing co-active imitative behaviors with profoundly mentally handicapped students. *Education and Training of the Mentally Retarded 20*, 260–67.

Sternberg, L., Pegnatore, L. & Hill, C. (1983). Establishing interactive communication behaviors with profoundly mentally handicapped students. *Journal of The Association for the Severely Handicapped 8*, 39–46.

Thompson, I. (1991). An academic-educative approach to behaviour problems. *NSW Journal of Special Education 14*, 16–22.

Thorndike, R.L., Hagen, E.P. & Sattler, J.M. (1986). *Stanford Binet Intelligence Scale* (4th edn). Chicago: Riverside Publishing Co.

van Dijk, J. (1986). An educational curriculum for deaf-blind multihandicapped persons. In D. Ellis (ed.), *Sensory impairments in mentally handicapped people*. London: Croom-Helm.

Wechsler, D. (1974). *Wechsler Intelligence Scale for Children — Revised*. New York: Psychological Corporation.

Williams, R. (1991). Choices, communication and control: A call for expanding them in the lives of people with severe disabilities. In L.H. Meyer, C.A. Peck & L. Brown (eds), *Critical issues in the lives of people with severe disabilities*. Baltimore: Paul H. Brookes.

Williams, W., Villa, R., Thousand, J. & Fox, W.L. (1989). Reader response: Is regular class placement really the issue? *Journal of The Association for Persons with Severe Handicaps 14 (4)*, 333–34.

Writer, J. (1987). A movement-based approach to the education of students who are sensory impaired/multihandicapped. In L. Goetz, D. Guess & K. Stremel-Campbell (eds), *Innovative program design for individuals with dual sensory impairments*. Baltimore: Paul H. Brookes.

York, J. & Rainforth, B. (1989). *Related educational services for individuals with severe disabilities: Report from the Related Services Subcommitteee of the TASH Critical Services Committee*. Seattle: The Association for Persons with Severe Handicaps.

York, J., Rainforth, B. & Dunn, W. (1990). Training needs of physical and occupational therapists who provide services to children and youth with severe disabilities. In A.P. Kaiser & C.M. McWhorter (eds), *Preparing personnel to work with persons with severe disabilities*. Baltimore: Paul H. Brookes.

Chapter 8

Enhancing Communication in Functional Settings: Putting Research into Practice

Nancy Butterfield and Ken Linfoot
Charles Sturt University-Mitchell
Bathurst, NSW

and

Michael Arthur
University of Newcastle
Newcastle, NSW

Previous chapters in this book have explored issues and presented research on features of the communicative behaviour of people with intellectual difficulties across a range of age groups and in many different settings. An important finding in many of those papers was that there are significant features of the contexts in which learners find themselves that may increase the likelihood that their behaviour is communicative. Conversely, there are other contextual features that may actually inhibit communicative behaviour.

This chapter provides some practical guidelines for the enhancement of communication skills in people with severe intellectual disabilities which have been developed from our findings about contextual effects on communication. As a result, the suggestions presented here derive from an ecological perspective, with consideration being given to our clients' ages, and are concerned with the encouragement of communication in naturally occurring environments rather than in artificial, or "training", settings. To this end, it is implicit that such strategies be implemented by all of the clients' likely communication partners. People such as parents, other relatives, teachers, teacher aides, and other professionals and caregivers working with the client can be helped to develop appropriate practical skills which will make the most of naturally occurring opportunities for communication. In this chapter, the term "communication partner" is used to refer broadly to any of these people, and the term "client" refers to individuals receiving their assistance.

While placing emphasis on the importance of social interaction to effective communication, this chapter also directs attention to the variety of forms of communication used by some students with intellectual disabilities. Some behaviours, which may have been dismissed as idiosyncratic, self-directed or maladaptive, are increasingly considered to serve some communicative purpose for the person concerned (Mirenda, Iacono & Williams, 1990; Burke, 1990; Doss & Reichle, 1989). Observation of clients and the people with whom they interact reveals that, in fact, such behaviours are often not noticed or responded to (Houghton, Bronicki & Guess, 1987). The task for communicative partners becomes one of learning to recognise and respond in an affirming manner to those communicative attempts.

To help prepare a wide variety of people to engage in communication-fostering interactions with those having intellectual disabilities, this chapter will:

1. provide an overview of functional communication and its development
2. present material on appropriate techniques for client and environmental assessment
3. present information on the considerations for programming
4. describe a series of instructional processes that can be implemented in the context of daily routines and selected according to the communicative level of the client.

Much of the material presented in this chapter is drawn from principles described in greater detail by Butterfield, Arthur, Linfoot & Sigafoos (in preparation) in a practical instructional manual for teachers of students with intellectual disabilities.

The Development of Functional Communication

Learning to communicate has been described in terms of three broad stages (Bates, Camaioni & Volterra, 1975; Bloom & Lahey, 1978; Dunst & Lowe, 1986; Harrison, Lombardino & Stapell, 1987; McLean & Snyder-McLean, 1987). Figure 8-1 illustrates the three broad stages of

<table>
<tr><th colspan="6">Learning to communicate</th></tr>
<tr><th colspan="4">Pre-verbal</th><th colspan="2">Verbal</th></tr>
<tr><td colspan="2">Pre-intentional
Primitive forms</td><td colspan="2">Intentional
Conventional forms</td><td colspan="2">Symbolic
Conventional use of symbolic forms</td></tr>
<tr><td colspan="2">Only those who frequently interact with the student may understand the behaviours.
The communication partner interprets the meaning of the behaviours.
Behaviours are idiosyncratic and non-conventional.
At first behaviours are not necessarily directed to a partner, and communication depends on those nearby interpreting what is required.
Later the behaviours are more often goal-directed and may be aimed at an object or partner. For example, staring at a required object and pointing, or gaining a partner's attention but not clearly indicating why.</td><td colspan="2">The student makes his or her intentions known to a partner.
The forms of behaviour used are increasingly mature. For example, the student may point to an object and use eye contact, or the student may take the partner's hand and place it on the object of interest.
More people are able to understand the purpose of the behaviours.
The communication process is now coordinated. The partner and the object of interest are encompassed by the one act. For example, eye gaze alternates from the object of interest to the person who is to receive the message.
There is combined use of vocalisations and gestures.
The student expects that the message will be understood and checks that this is so. If not, the behaviour may escalate.
Satisfaction is apparent when the student's needs are met.</td><td colspan="2">The symbolic system may be words, signs or pictures.
Symbolic forms are now used to carry out the functions previously achieved by non-verbal means.
Initially the student refers to items, people or events present at the time (in context).
The student progresses to using the symbolic system to refer to items, people or events not present at the time (out of context).
The student may use a multi-modal system of symbols and/or gestures and/or vocalisations.
Symbols can be combined to extend the syntactic structure of the system used.</td></tr>
<tr><td>Idiosyncratic behaviours</td><td>Goal-directed behaviour</td><td>Convention-al gestures</td><td>Early words (actions, functional behaviour)</td><td>First words, context-dependent</td><td>Reference to out-of-context events</td></tr>
</table>

Figure 8-1: The continuum representing the process of learning to communicate.
(Adapted from Bates, Camaoini & Volterra, 1975; Bloom & Lahey, 1978; McLean & Snyder-McLean, 1978; Dunst & Lowe, 1986: In N. Butterfield, 1993, p 2)

communication development, including both pre-verbal and verbal communication. An expanded description of each stage is also provided. Given that people with severe intellectual disabilities are reported to have difficulty in developing the conventional modes of communication, it is proposed that attention be given to the development of pre-verbal abilities, prior to learning a symbolic system (Reichle, York & Sigafoos, 1991).

For some clients, social or interactive behaviour may be described as "pre-intentional". That is, the individual does not clearly indicate a particular communicative intent by the behaviour used, but the communication partner interprets what may be intended. For example, crying in the presence of a dropped toy, or when a nappy is wet, may be interpreted as a call for attention to that situation. The behaviours used at this stage are typically idiosyncratic and often are only understood by those who frequently interact with the infant or young child. Later in the pre-intentional stage, behaviours can be identified as goal-directed, where the child focuses specifically on the object of interest, may vocalise and gesture toward this but does not demonstrate an awareness of the adult as a communication partner or as a tool to assist in achieving the goal.

Intentional behaviours are those in which the individual shows a coordination between attention to an object and awareness of the instrumental role of the communication partner. In addition, the individual demonstrates an expectation that his or her intent will be understood (Sugarman, 1984; Dunst & Lowe, 1986; McLean & Snyder-McLean, 1987). More people can read or understand the behaviours as communicative, as the gestures used are more conventional, such as pointing. Early words typically appear toward the end of this stage, when a person is learning to talk.

The client is now a functional communicator, displaying the ability to interact with a partner for a set purpose. It is typical to begin then to use a symbolic system rather than gestures to achieve the same functional ends. The symbolic system usually consists of speech; however, the use of a signing or pictorial system can augment speech or act as an alternative to speech. As use of the symbolic system matures, the client is able to refer to objects not immediately present, resulting in increased power to interact with others in the environment.

In addition to recognising the stage of the communication process, caregivers also need to recognise the functions intended by the behaviours. The function intended is the purpose of the communicative behaviour, which may include requesting assistance, objects or attention; greetings and farewells; responding to one's name; protesting; and requesting information about objects or events. Mastery of these functional aspects of communication by the student underpins social interaction. The achievement of functional communication may be evident at each of the stages of communication development, with individuals varying in the maturity and complexity of forms used (Butterfield, 1991).

The development of functional communication in a student with an intellectual disability involves two considerations. Attention must be paid, first, to the student's starting point in the continuum of learning to communicate (Figure 8-1) and, second, to the nature of the functions that the student is able to master in purposeful interactions. If realistic goals are to be set for increasing communicative competence, then these factors need to be jointly considered before selecting and implementing intervention procedures.

Client and Environmental Assessment

The purpose of assessment is to identify goals for the interventions or procedures used to help the client develop communicative behaviours. In the light of what has been said so far, it will be clear that assessment will need to focus on the communicative functions used by the individual, the forms used to achieve those functions and the person's social interaction skills in various settings and with different people.

The Caregiver Interview

The caregiver interview is a first step to learning about the student's communication abilities. A format for the interview appears in the instructional manual by Butterfield, Arthur, Linfoot & Sigafoos (in preparation). The interview includes the following areas of inquiry:

1. The client's motor and sensory abilities
2. The client's primary communication mode, and how easy it is to understand; the identification of a preferred mode of communication for the future
3. Activities which encourage/discourage interaction with the client
4. The client's likes/dislikes
5. The behaviours the client uses to achieve a range of communicative functions, and the context in which they occur
6. The behaviours the client uses to demonstrate a range of social skills, and the context in which they occur.

The information obtained from the interview provides a basis for identifying the forms of behaviour used by the client to achieve a communicative end and a profile of the pragmatic functions and social skills demonstrated by the client. From this, the following conclusions can be drawn:

1. The stage at which the client is functioning in terms of the continuum of pre-intentional, intentional and symbolic levels of communication
2. The functional abilities that may need development
3. The social skills that may need to be extended.

The planning of intervention strategies is inherently linked to this information.

The ABC

To support these judgements of the caregiver, it is recommended that careful observations are made of the client's behaviours in a variety of settings and during various activities. Using the Antecedent Behaviour Consequent (ABC) format (Wolery, Bailey & Sugai, 1988, pp 356–59), a record is made of the specific *behaviours* of the student, the events that occur in that environment immediately before (*antecedent to*) the behaviour and the events that occur immediately following (*consequent to*) the behaviour. The analysis of this information can demonstrate possible relationships between an individual's (communicative) behaviour and other events, either stimuli or reinforcers, in the environment. This process allows those who interact with the client in a variety of settings to increase their awareness of not only the behaviours that are communicative, but also any of their own behaviours that may hinder or assist the communication process. In addition, it may highlight a difference in interaction with the client across settings and personnel.

Communication Partner Skills

The fact that communication is a two-way process highlights the need for a balanced view of assessment. Not only should a client's communication abilities be assessed, but also the abilities of the communication partner to recognise and respond to the client's attempts at communication. Communication partners in all settings need to reflect on their own interactions with the client in a self-critical way so that personal goals that will increase the interactive nature of the setting can be identified. For example, partners should consider whether they:

1. look for opportunities to promote interaction
2. adjust routines to allow time for interaction
3. anticipate clients' needs and thus eliminate their need to communicate
4. talk to the students about daily routines as they proceed
5. pause in routines so that clients have time to respond

6. ensure that opportunities for making choices are provided to clients across activities.

Assessment is therefore a three-phase process, involving an interview with a caregiver, observation of the client and reflection by the communication partner on his or her ability to foster an interactive environment. An analysis of the material collected using these three techniques will need to address the extent to which the client's behaviour is functional, the contextual features that are associated with the client's communicative behaviour and the nature or readability of the communication forms used.

Considerations for Programming

From the analysis of the nature of the communicative exchanges with the client, caregivers have an opportunity to make some decisions about programming objectives.

The initial goal for the learner may be to establish a desire to be communicative and a realisation of the power that communicating has to increase his or her control over the environment in which interaction occurs. In addition, the client may need to develop increased responsiveness in social settings, an understanding of turn-taking in communicative interactions, and an ability to make goals known to a communication partner by displaying intentional behaviours.

The next goal will be the selection of a vocabulary to be learned. This will need to be done with a view to helping the client use the language functions and social interaction skills that are personally relevant. The most powerful vocabulary usually includes items that represent the concepts, functions and skills in which the client has already expressed an interest and which are related to the client's environmental demands. Vocabulary items should also be related to a particular client's needs in future situations, such as a regular education placement option, community-living arrangement or workplace setting. Further discussion of issues related to vocabulary selection appears in Chapter 4.

When a particular individual is not able to be best assisted to communicate by relying on verbal means, some attention will need to be given to the selection of an alternative communication mode or system. For some clients, learning how to make the best use of gestures or facial or vocal expressions may be the most appropriate initial aim. For others, a symbolic system may be within their repertoire or able to be introduced. At all times these decisions need to be made in consultation with the multidisciplinary team responsible for the client's individual programming needs, including parents and caregivers.

Bloomberg and Johnson (1991) describe a continuum of communication systems, progressing from the least to the most abstract. "Unaided" systems include all procedures used to communicate that do not require hardware usage. For example, facial expression, body language, pointing, using natural gestures, mime, signing, fingerspelling or speech. "Aided" systems are those using some object or means of production external to the student and include objects, miniatures, pictures, photographs, line drawings, symbol systems, and the printed word and spelling.

The most significant step in deciding what to teach individuals is the analysis of their daily activities for communication opportunities. This can highlight the functions the client needs to master and the social skills appropriate to each situation. It can help to identify when the client needs to communicate and what he or she needs to communicate. Problems such as the unhelpful anticipation of a client's needs and timing inappropriate for interaction with the client can be identified.

In addition to analysing an activity to identify programming goals, possible ways to increase the communicative opportunities during this activity can also be identified by asking the following kinds of questions:

1. Can access to an object or to the activity be blocked so that the client needs to ask for assistance?
2. Is it possible to increase the opportunities for making choices within the activity?
3. Can preferred or needed items be hidden or placed out of reach?
4. Can an inappropriate object be offered instead of the item needed for the activity in order to elicit protesting behaviour?

The context of daily activities therefore provides the basis for the instructional setting, with the goals of instruction being based on the needs of the client as identified in the assessment process, and on the communicative demands of the activity. Cipani (1991) has identified a series of language development activities for very young children, which focuses on everyday self-care activities such as meal preparation, brushing teeth, washing and grooming, dressing, bath time, playing with toys and household cleaning. Using a mastery learning format, Cipani shows how objectives such as requesting skills, beginning conversations, vocabulary recognition and expressive skills can be developed during those activities in naturalistic and functional settings. For other learners, contexts in which self-care, residential, recreational or work activities occur would also be appropriate. Calculator and Jorgensen (1991) highlight the need for programming objectives to truly reflect the functional demands of the interactive setting rather than being based on relatively abstract concept development such as matching symbols with objects. Programming steps can therefore be summarised as follows:

1. Review the client's daily activities in order to identify the opportunities for communication
2. Set objectives relative to the client's level of communicative abilities and to the functional demands of the activity
3. Identify personal goals for the communication partner
4. Look for opportunities to generate increased communication attempts from the client
5. Decide on an instructional process that will best match the objective and functional level of the client (see next section)
6. Implement the program in the context of daily activities
7. Monitor the client's progress
8. Evaluate and review the program.

Linking Instruction with Assessment and Programming

The other important outcome of assessment is to identify the level at which instruction is likely to be most appropriate and, consequently, to identify the most suitable instructional techniques. Butterfield, Arthur, Linfoot & Sigafoos (in preparation) have summarised instructional strategies from research on communication disorders in students with intellectual disabilities and linked these with the continuum of communicative behaviour development (pre-intentional, intentional and symbolic communication) discussed earlier in this chapter. All strategies recommended stress the importance of naturalistic instructional settings.

Pre-intentional to Intentional Communication

For the client operating at the pre-intentional level, the main objectives will be to increase the client's responsiveness in the social setting and to develop the partner's ability to read and respond to behaviours as if they are communicative. The reinforcing nature of such interactions will assist in the development of increasingly intentional behaviours. With the development of intentional behaviour, the range of people who understand the client's actions is increased, so that there is a greater match between what is expressed and its impact on life's experiences. Table 8-1 lists the strategies suitable for achieving the objectives typically needed by individuals at this level. Siegel-Causey and Guess (1989) and Harrison, Lombardino and Stapell (1987) are particularly valuable sources of further information.

Table 8-1: Instructional strategies recommended for developing pre-intentional to intentional communication abilities. (Arthur & Butterfield, 1993, p 9)

Strategy	Purpose
Contingent responding (MacDonald & Gillette, 1984)	The student learns to make an "if . . . then" association between the production of a vocal or motor behaviour and some form of consequence. This highlights the importance of the communication partner responding consistently to behaviours that may be reflexive, as if they are in fact communicative.
Wait and signal (MacDonald & Gillette, 1984)	The student learns that there is a turn-taking and joint attention role associated with social or other interactive routines. The communication partner can pause in the process of normal routines and games, before making eye contact with the student to signal the expectation of a response. Student responses are then reinforced in socially and functionally appropriate ways.
Shaping (Harrison, Lombardino & Stapell, 1987)	The student is reinforced for using successively closer approximations of a new form of communication. Thus the communication partner may respond to the student's whinges by suggesting that the student "ask" for help, before modelling eye contact and smiling. As the student incorporates approximations of these communicative forms, assistance is offered and reinforcement delivered.
Referencing (Bruce, 1983; McLean & Snyder-McLean, 1978)	The communication partner directs and redirects the student's attention to the object of interest and the communication partner. The student learns to communicate goals to a partner. For example, the student may be staring at a desired object and vocalising. Assistance can be given to direct the student to look at the partner as well as the object.

Intentional to Symbolic Communication

The following strategies are designed to help the client who is at the intentional level, to develop symbolic communicative behaviours. Examples of this communicative form include speech, pictures, photographs, objects or a combination of these. The strategies are designed to be implemented in the context of daily activities, so that contextually relevant vocabulary is introduced and the functional aspect of communication is stressed. A summary of these strategies is presented in Table 8-2. It should be noted that, in order to increase the need for communication, strategies that involve discrete changes in the learning environment may be used (blocking access, placing objects out of reach, offering objects out of context).

Extending Symbolic Abilities

Here the focus is on increasing the client's understanding of the use of a symbol as a means of communication in an expanding set of environments. While some table-top caregiver instruction may be necessary to extend conceptual awareness of symbolic use, client use of the symbols in a variety of environments is the key. Instruction should always extend to daily application for functional purposes.

Table 8-2: Instructional strategies recommended for developing intentional to symbolic communication abilities. (Arthur & Butterfield, 1993, pp 10–11)

Strategy	Purpose
Mand-model (Rogers-Warren & Warren, 1980)	The communication partner, after noticing the student's interest in an object or event, initiates the interaction, mands (requests) a response and models the required response if necessary. The student is assisted through the process of learning to use a symbolic system in response to a request. For example, a student may go to the cupboard and take out the cordial bottle, indicating a desire for a drink. The communication partner notices the request, models the use of an appropriate symbol and asks the student to respond, by saying, "Tell me what you want."
Time delay (Halle, Baer & Spradlin, 1981; Schwartz, Anderson & Halle, 1989)	By pausing in a well-known activity for a set time and indicating by non-verbal means that a response is expected, the communication partner assists the student to increase the spontaneous use of newly learned behaviours. Continuation of the activity acts to reinforce the communication attempt. Avoiding providing verbal cues is a key to the effectiveness of this strategy in generating the desire to initiate communicative exchanges in the student.
Interrupted behaviour chain (Alwell, Hunt, Goetz & Sailor, 1989)	Students are motivated to request objects or assistance when a well-known routine is interrupted and an out-of-context item is inserted into the activity. The student should be familiar with the activity and have a strong desire to want to complete the task. For example, after beginning the activity of tooth-cleaning the communication partner removes the toothpaste, places the appropriate symbol in view and indicates that the student is to make a request for the item in order to complete cleaning the teeth. The activity continues only if the student responds appropriately. If not, no reinforcement is given and the process returns to the beginning steps in the task.
Incidental teaching (Hart & Risley, 1986; Warren & Kaiser, 1986)	Once the student is able to initiate an interaction, it is possible to encourage the use of expanded forms using the procedure of increasing the complexity of verbal prompts. A natural prompt such as "What do you want?" can be used in the first instance to elicit a response. If no response is offered, the communication partner can add, "You need to tell me what you want", and finally, if necessary, can add the request for the student to say "want...".

Table 8-3 describes the strategies that may be implemented for clients at this level.

Summary

This chapter has provided a glimpse into the application of research findings to the varying contexts in which communication instruction most effectively occurs. Three concluding points are salient.

First, communication must be viewed as a transactional process. No

Table 8-3: Instructional strategies recommended for extending symbolic abilities. (Arthur & Butterfield, 1993, p 12)

Strategy	Purpose
Verbal prompt-free (Mirenda & Dattilo, 1987)	The student gains access to an item/event by touching its symbol either accidentally or purposefully. Physical prompts may be given, but no verbal cues are delivered. If the student touches the symbol, verbal acknowledgment can accompany access to the item. The symbol may be in the form of a line drawing, photograph or miniature. This strategy lends itself well to the selection of a leisure activity. For example, the student can make a choice between watching a video, making a milkshake, playing with a ball or jumping on the trampoline.
Generalised request/reject (Keogh & Reichle, 1985; Reichle, York & Sigafoos, 1991).	Generic symbols are selected to indicate request (such as a happy face) and reject (such as a sad face). The use of symbols for these functions may be necessary for students who have a range of other symbols that they are able to use in communicative exchanges, and who need to link these symbols with such generic functions as request, reject and provide information. For example, if a student points to the picture of "sandwich", this may be to request, reject or to tell you about a sandwich. The use of the symbol, to indicate the function, accompanied by the object label can expand the functional power of the symbol system.
Match to sample (Thorley, Jardine & Binepal, 1984)	Using the principles of discrimination learning, the student establishes a clear concept for a given symbol. This strategy is based on massed trials and the careful control of discriminative features in stimuli. It can therefore provide the opportunity to increase the student's conceptual understanding and use of symbols across settings, time and personnel. For example, the student may visit the bowling alley once a week, and so practice in using symbols associated with this activity may be needed between visits.

longer should communication interventions be considered a one-way process or be confined to a training paradigm. How we interact as communication partners is as important as our systematic use of strategies designed to stimulate participation by our clients, a point underlined by the findings of researchers such as Houghton, Bronicki and Guess (1987).

Second, the continuum of communicative behaviours allows for the dynamic use of any of the instructional strategies as appropriate to the needs and contexts of the learner. The levels simply suggest a starting point, and programs will benefit from the active monitoring of individual progress.

Finally, communication programming and instruction must be actively pursued. To label communication simply as a cross-curricular concern without systematically planning for change is to abdicate responsibility in an area that is arguably the cornerstone for much other learning in the lives of students with intellectual disabilities.

References

Alwell, M., Hunt, P., Goetz, L. & Sailor, W. (1989). Teaching generalized communicative behaviors within interrupted behavior chain contexts. *Journal of The Association for Persons with Severe Handicaps 14*, 91–100.

Arthur, M. & Butterfield, N. (1993) Creating Communicative Contexts: An Australian Study. Paper presented to the 1993 Annual Conference of The Association for Persons with Severe Handicaps, November, Chicago. USA.

Bates, E., Camaioni, L. & Volterra, V. (1975). The acquisition of performatives prior to speech. *Merrill-Palmer Quarterly 21*, 205–26.

Bloom, L. & Lahey, M. (1978). *Language development and language disorders*. New York: John Wiley & Sons.

Bloomberg, K. & Johnson, H. (1991). *Communication without speech*. Melbourne: ACER.

Bruner, J. (1983) Child's talk: Learning to use language. New York: Norton.

Burke, G.M. (1990). Unconventional behavior: A communicative interpretation in individuals with severe disabilities. *Topics in Language Disorders 10*, 75–85.

Butterfield, N. (1991). Assessment of preverbal communicative abilities in students with severe intellectual disability. *Australia and New Zealand Journal of Developmental Disabilities 17 (4)*, 347–64.

Butterfield, N. (1993). Merging developmental and functional emphases. A discussion of issues in communication programming for students with severe intellectual disabilities. In Quality and Equality Proceedings of the ASSID National Conference, University of Newcastle, Australia.

Butterfield, N., Arthur, M., Linfoot, K. & Sigafoos, G. (in preparation). *Communication across contexts*.

Calculator, S.N. & Jorgensen, C.M. (1991). Integrating AAC instruction into regular education settings: Expounding on best practices. *Augmentative and Alternative Communication 7*, 204–11.

Cipani, E. (ed.) (1991). *A guide to developing language competence in preschool children with severe and moderate handicaps*. Springfield: Charles C. Thomas.

Doss, S. & Reichle, J. (1989). Establishing communicative alternatives to the emission of socially motivated excess behavior: A review. *Journal of The Association for Persons with Severe Handicaps 14 (2)*, 101–12.

Dunst, C.J. & Lowe, L.W. (1986). From reflex to symbol: Describing, explaining and fostering communicative competence. *Augmentative and Alternative Communication 2*, 11–18.

Halle, J.W., Baer, D.M. & Spradlin, J.E. (1981). Teachers' generalized use of delay as a stimulus control procedure to increase language use in handicapped children. *Journal of Applied Behavior Analysis 14*, 389–409.

Harrison, J., Lombardino, L.J. & Stapell, J.B. (1987). The development of early communication: Using developmental literature for selecting communication goals. *The Journal of Special Education 20*, 463–73.

Hart, B.M. & Risley, T.R. (1986). Establishing use of descriptive adjectives in the spontaneous speech of disadvantaged preschool children. *Journal of Applied Behavior Analysis 1*, 109–20.

Houghton, J., Bronicki, B. & Guess, D. (1987). Opportunities to express preferences and make choices among students with severe disabilities in classroom settings. *Journal of The Association for Persons with Severe Handicaps 12 (1)*, 18–27.

Keogh, W. & Reichle, J. (1985). Communication intervention for the "difficult to teach" severely handicapped. In S. Warren & A. Rogers-Warren (eds), *Teaching functional language*. Baltimore: University Park Press.

MacDonald, J.D. & Gillette, Y. (1984) Ecomaps: A manual for assessing language through conversation. Columbus, OH: Ohio State University Research Foundation.

McLean, J. & Snyder-McLean, L. (1978). A transactional approach to early language training. Columbus, OH.: Charles E. Merrill.

McLean, J. & Snyder-McLean, L. (1987). Form and function of communicative behaviour among persons with severe developmental disabilities. *Australia and New Zealand Journal of Developmental Disabilities 13*, 83–98.

Mirenda, P. & Dattilo, J. (1987). Instructional techniques in alternative communication for students with severe intellectual handicaps. *Augmentative and Alternative Communication 3*, 143–52.

Mirenda, P., Iacono, T. & Williams, R. (1990). Communication options for persons with severe and profound disabilities: State of the art and future directions. *Journal of The Association for Persons with Severe Handicaps 15*, 3–21.

Reichle, J., York, J. & Sigafoos, J. (1991). *Implementing augmentative and alternative communication: Strategies for learners with severe disabilities*. Baltimore: Paul H. Brookes.

Rogers-Warren, A. & Warren, S. (1980). Mands for verbalization: Facilitating the display of newly trained language in children. *Behavior Modification 4*, 361–82.

Schwartz, I.S., Anderson, S.R. & Halle, J.W. (1989). Training teachers to use naturalistic time delay: Effects on teacher behavior and on the language use of students. *Journal of The Association for Persons with Severe Handicaps 14*, 48–57.

Siegel-Causey, E. & Guess, D. (1989). *Enhancing nonsymbolic communication interactions among learners with severe disabilities*. Baltimore: Paul H. Brookes.

Sugarman, S. (1984). The development of preverbal communicative competence. In R.L. Schiefelbusch & S. Pickar (eds), *Communicative competence: Acquisition and intervention*. Baltimore: University Park Press.

Thorley, B., Jardine, J. & Binepal, T. (1984). *North Rocks Project: The concept program: Teaching skills in discrimination and classification to severely handicapped children*. Sydney: Macquarie University Special Education Centre.

Warren, S.F. & Kaiser, A.P. (1986). Incidental language teaching: A critical review. *Journal of Speech and Hearing Disorders 51*, 291–99.

Wolery, M., Bailey, D.B. & Sugai, G.M. (1988). *Effective teaching principles and practices of Applied Behavior Analysis with exceptional children*. Boston: Allyn & Bacon.

Index